MANUAL OF PERITONEAL DIALYSIS

Distributors

for the United States and Canada: Kluwer Academic Publishers, PO Box 358, Accord Station, Hingham, MA 02018-0358, USA
for all other countries: Kluwer Academic Publishers Group, Distribution Center, PO Box 322, 3300 AH Dordrecht, The Netherlands

British Library Cataloguing in Publication Data

Coles, G.A.
  Manual of peritoneal dialysis.
  1. Man. Kidneys. Peritoneal dialysis
  I. Title
  617.461059

  ISBN 0-7462-0081-1

Copyright

Published in the United Kingdom by Kluwer Academic Publishers, PO Box 55, Lancaster, UK.

Kluwer Academic Publishers BV incorporates the publishing programmes of D. Reidel, Martinus Nijhoff, Dr W. Junk and MTP Press.

Printed and bound in Great Britain by Butler and Tanner Ltd., Frome and London.

MANUAL OF PERITONEAL DIALYSIS

Practical Procedures for Medical and Nursing Staff

G. A. Coles

Consultant Physician
Department of Renal Medicine
University of Wales College of Medicine
Cardiff Royal Infirmary
Newport Road
Cardiff, Wales, UK

KLUWER ACADEMIC PUBLISHERS

DORDRECHT - BOSTON - LONDON

Contents

Introduction

Peritoneal dialysis (PD) is in widespread use for the treatment of acute and chronic renal failure. A considerable amount of knowledge about the various procedures and problems associated with this form of treatment has accumulated over recent years, particularly since the introduction of continuous ambulatory peritoneal dialysis (CAPD). However to date the information regarding the more technical or practical aspects of PD has been largely scattered in various books and journals. There appears to be no straightforward text concerned with these points suitable for recommending to junior doctors or nurses dealing with patients receiving this therapy. Though in-house-training is of considerable value it takes time and I have noticed that on a number of occasions in our own unit, technical problems with PD have not been dealt with quickly because of lack of knowledge in the staff on duty. There thus appeared to me to be a need for a short book giving firm advice on how to perform the various procedures and how to deal with problems as they arose. This manual is an attempt to fulfil that aim. Initially it was tried and tested on the renal unit in the Cardiff Royal Infirmary for 3 years. Prior to publishing it has been extensively revised and updated.

The information presented here has been obtained partly from the literature but also from personal experience of temporary PD for more than 21 years, long-term PD for 11 years and the management of some 260 CAPD patients over the last 8 years. The text is deliberately dogmatic in places as I felt that junior medical and nursing staff when faced with a problem wanted firm, practical advice and not a long balanced discussion. Thus detailed explanations as to why certain steps are necessary have been avoided deliberately. However where there is a genuine uncertainty as to the best course of action I have made this plain.

Many of the procedures described can be performed by trained nurses but where I felt a doctor should be responsible I have indicated this by the letter D alongside the relevant heading.

The manual is divided into two sections. Section A describes the techniques and problems involved with temporary PD. It is particularly concerned with the use of the Trocath cannula together with a Y type tubing set and drainage bag. However other cannulae need to be managed in a similar way. Section B deals with long-term PD using the Tenckhoff double cuff Silastic catheter. Again alternative permanent peritoneal cannulae require similar procedures. In this text the words catheter and cannula are used in an interchangeable manner.

The book does not concern itself with the indications for dialysis nor the more general management of renal failure. A further reading list on PD itself is given at the end of the text.

This work is therefore offered in the hope that it will prove useful to medical and nursing staff in district general hospitals performing occasional PD as well as to specialised renal units to aid them in training new personnel.

Acknowledgements

I am grateful to the nursing staff of the Renal Unit, Cardiff Royal Infirmary and in particular Sister Georgina Hourahane, Sister in charge of the CAPD Unit for many helpful suggestions and contributions to this manual. Mr D Roberts and Miss T Richards, past and present renal pharmacists, assisted with the assessment of drug dosage and handling. My medical colleagues, especially Professor A W Asscher, Dr D J Fisher and Dr J D Williams, have kindly provided advice but any mistakes or inadequacies are my own. Miss K Shepherd, Mrs W Thomas and Miss R Sultana valiantly typed the several versions of this manuscript. Dr P L Clarke and the staff of MTP Press Ltd have made publication of this manual possible and I acknowledge their advice and help with gratitude. Finally I am grateful to my wife and family for considerable forbearance and encouragement.

Section A

TEMPORARY PERITONEAL DIALYSIS

Introduction

This section is concerned with peritoneal dialysis using in particular the Trocath rigid cannula. All the techniques associated with the dialysis procedure are described together with comments on the common problems which can occur. The index lists the subject headings. The advice given is often duplicated but this has been done deliberately as in practice a problem may present in more than one way.

Index for Section A

Oedema of abdominal skin
Oedema of genitalia
Dehydration
Hypotension
Hypertension
Ascites
Hypoalbuminaemia
Obesity
Dialysis after laparotomy
Ileus, obstruction, adhesions
Colostomy, ileostomy,
    ureterostomy, conduit
Abdominal fistulae and drains
Blood urea does not fall

Disequilibrium
Hyperkalaemia
Hypokalaemia
Hyperglycaemia
Hypercalcaemia
Chest complications
Air under diaphragm
Hernia
Choice of cycle volume
Dwell times
Continuous or intermittent dialysis
Choice of fluid
Heating of fluid
Automatic machines

Choice of cannula   D

There are at least three types of cannulae suitable for temporary peritoneal dialysis (Figure A1)

1. The Trocath cannula. The technique of insertion is described in detail in this manual. The advantages of this cannula are that it can be inserted easily at the bedside and the procedure is relatively quick. Furthermore large cycle volumes can be used straight away, i.e. 1 or 2 litres. The main disadvantages are that it is subject to movement and is increasingly liable to infection the longer it remains in place. It is also sometimes uncomfortable for the patient.

2. An acute Tenckhoff cannula. This consists of a Silastic tube with a single Dacron cuff. The technique for insertion is identical to that described in Section B of this manual but the Dacron cuff lies close to the skin exit site. There is no inner cuff to be placed just above the peritoneum. The major advantage of this cannula is that after the first week of usage it is much less likely to get infected. The disadvantages are that cycle volumes will initially have to be low, e.g. 500 ml for most adults, to reduce the chances of leakage. This may mean less efficient dialysis. Furthermore removal involves cutting down over the cuff and freeing it before the cannula itself can be withdrawn. Details on usage of Silastic catheters are presented in Section B.

3. A Seldinger type cannula. William Cook make a cannula which is inserted using a Seldinger technique. In brief a needle is inserted into the abdomen and a guide wire is threaded through the lumen. The needle is withdrawn and the cannula is passed over the wire which is then removed. The advantage is that the cannula dilates the tract itself so that the skin and subcutaneous tissues are tight around it minimising the chances of leakage and subsequent infection. The disadvantage is that it may prove difficult to insert the cannula if the tissues provide much resistance. Furthermore as currently supplied the set is not suitable for relatively obese patients.

In the author's opinion if dialysis is likely to be relatively short lived and/or needs to be efficient from the start then the Trocath is preferable as it is relatively easy and quick to insert. Furthermore junior medical staff can be taught the technique with little difficulty. If however dialysis is likely to be prolonged, i.e. 2 weeks or more, then a Silastic catheter is preferred but insertion takes longer and more skill is required. Training of medical staff similarly takes longer.

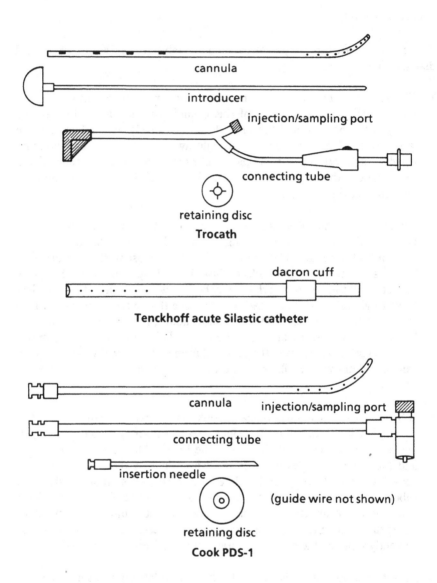

Figure A1 Temporary PD catheters

Trolley setting for cannulation

1. Clean top and bottom shelves and sides of trolley with detergent, then sterilise with isopropyl alcohol 70% (Sterets Alcowipe).

2. Leave top shelf free of equipment.

3. *Bottom Shelf*
   Sterile gown
   Sterile gloves (2 pairs of correct size)
   Theatre masks (disposable)
   Theatre caps (disposable)
   Povidone-iodine in alcohol
   Chlorhexidine 1:200 (Hibitane)
   Suture pack
   Fenestration drape or cystoscopy sheet
   Sterile 4" x 4" swabs - 2 packets of 5 each
   Peritoneal dialysis trocar and cannula
   15 gauge long needle
   No. 11 scalpel
   Lignocaine 2% plain x 10 ml
   Syringes 10 ml x 1
   Needles, green x 2, blue x 2, orange x 2 (gauges 21, 23, 25)
   Sutures, either 3/0 328 or 2/0 667
   Elastoplast strapping (new box)
   Micropore 1" (new roll) or alternative adhesive tape
   Disposable dressing bag (attached below top shelf, right side)
   Bag for reusable items (attached below top shelf, left side)

4. *At the bedside*
   a. Drip stand.
   b. Two litres of heated dialysate solution and required additives, run through a Y type peritoneal dialysis giving set. (Leave sterile cover attached to end.)
   c. Drainage bag attached to bed.
   d. Large polythene measuring jar, marked with the patient's name.
   e. Observation charts and peritoneal dialysis record chart.
   f. Tray containing 2 and 5 ml syringes, 21 gauge needles, nonsterile gloves, alcohol wipes and a selection of additives. Cover tray with a dressing towel and clearly mark with patient's name.
   g. Tray on floor for placing under drainage bag. One universal container half-filled with povidone-iodine to be placed in this tray.

5

Peritoneal dialysis cannulation for the nurse (Figure A2)

1. Help explain the procedure to the patient, together with the doctor.
2. Screen the bed and ask the patient to micturate.
3. Lay the patient in a semi-recumbent position on two pillows and shave the abdomen if necessary.
4. Put face mask on patient.
5. Nurse puts mask on, washes hands and brings trolley to the bedside.
6. Expose patient's abdomen, keeping the rest of the body warm.
7. Open all packs as per aseptic technique procedure. Before breaking open lignocaine ampoules, swab the ampoule necks with alcohol wipes.
8. After the doctor has inserted the cannula, the Y type giving set is connected by the nurse to the sterile extension (without contamination). The nurse commences the dialysate flow.
9. After free flow in and out of the abdomen has been established, the cannula is sutured into position and the nurse helps cut layers of clean elastoplast for the dressing. The dressing should be applied by the doctor.
10. *The nurse should ensure that the connecting tube is strapped* to the abdomen, freeing it from kinking and pulling to avoid disconnection and leakage.
11. Before leaving the patient, sit him upright in bed, if possible, and make him comfortable. A bed cradle may be used to relieve pressure on the abdomen.
12. Record observations of temperature, pulse and blood pressure and commence peritoneal dialysis chart.
13. Observe rate of dialysis flow and colour of fluid.
14. Remove trolley from bedside and clear away equipment. Wash the trolley.
15. Wash hands.

Insertion of cannula   D

1. Unless patient unconscious, *doctor* to explain to patient beforehand reason for and nature of peritoneal dialysis.
2. If necessary, sedate patient with diazepam.
3. Patient to empty bladder. If unconscious, catheterise aseptically and leave catheter in until after procedure completed. Doctor must confirm empty bladder by percussion.
4. Shave abdomen.

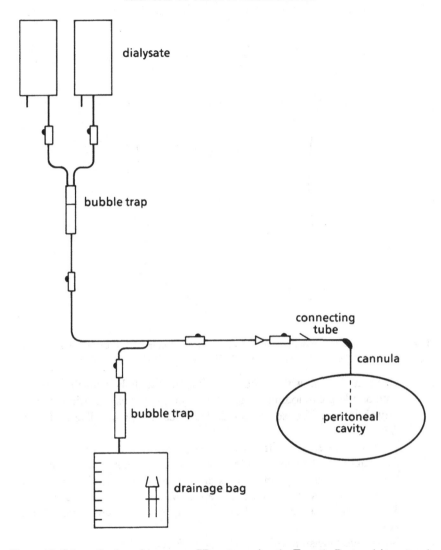

Figure A2 Schematic view of temporary PD system using the Trocath, Baxter giving set and drainage bag

5.   Set up prewarmed fluid (2 x 1 litre) containing 500 units of heparin per litre. Run through the Y-giving set and attach sterile drainage bag. Hang the fresh dialysate from a drip stand and the drainage bag from the side of the bed. Keep sterile cover over patient end of tubing.

6.   Doctor to wear mask and hat. Other staff to wear masks. Doctor to scrub, gown and glove up.

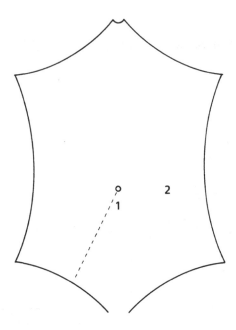

Figure A3.1 Sites for temporary PD cannula. 1 = Preferred sub-umbilical site; 2 = Alternative flank approach; - - - - - = Approximate course of inferior epigastric artery

7. Clean abdomen with povidone-iodine or alcoholic chlorhexidine if patient allergic to iodine. Patient to be lying as flat as condition allows.

8. Dry abdomen. Choose site about 3 to 6 cm below umbilicus. (Figure A3.1)

9. Infiltrate chosen site with local anaesthetic, penetrating vertically up to full length of 21 gauge needle depending on patient's size. Pull hard back on syringe at point of maximum penetration. If air comes into syringe the bowel has been perforated. Withdraw needle and discard. Try at a fresh site at least 2 cm either up or down linea alba. (Figure A3.2)

10. Make *small* incision with No. 11 blade. (Figure A3.3)

11. Insert cannula with introducer inside through skin (Figure A3.4). The black marks on the cannula should face the patient's feet. Ask patient to lift head and put the chin on the chest thus tensing the abdominal muscles.

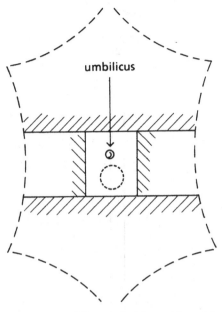

Figure A3.2 Insertion of temporary PD cannula. The position of the sterile towels on the abdomen is shown. The dotted circle represents the area to be anaesthetized approximately 4 cm diameter

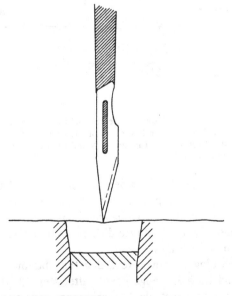

Figure A3.3 Vertical incision with a No.11 blade

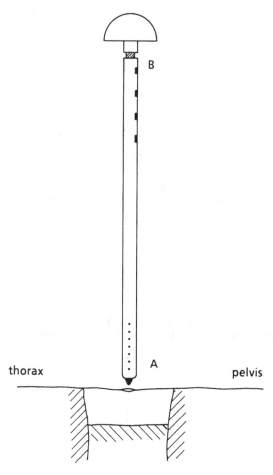

Figure A3.4 Trocath assembled and about to be inserted into the incision. Note the sharp end of the introducer protruding from the lower end of the cannula. The black marks are facing the pelvis. One hand should steady the cannula at A and the other should advance and rotate the handle of the introducer, B

12. Advance cannula controlling penetration with one hand at skin level. A twisting motion aids penetration. In some patients two levels of resistance are felt, the linea alba and the peritoneum itself. Once inside the peritoneal cavity resistance disappears and if any fluid is present it will be seen in the catheter.

13. Some nephrologists advocate filling the abdomen with one litre of dialysis fluid via a 15 gauge needle after step 10. If this technique is used the operator must avoid touching the giving set.

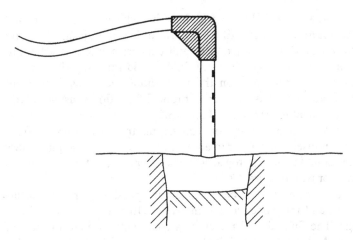

Figure A3.5 Filling the abdomen with PD fluid via the connecting tube prior to placement of the cannula in the pelvis

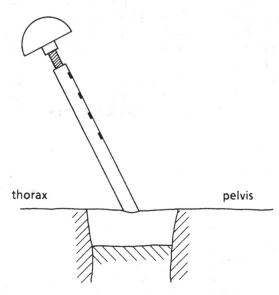

thorax   pelvis

Figure A3.6 The cannula is being advanced into the pelvis. Note the introducer has been pulled back so that the sharp point no longer protrudes from the internal end. The black marks are facing the pelvis

14. Once cannula is in abdomen withdraw introducer about 2 cm and advance cannula until all the side holes are judged to be intraperitoneal. Remove introducer and connect connecting tube. Fill abdomen with one or two litres of fluid. Avoid touching giving set. If cannula is in correct position the fluid should go in as a constant stream. If the cannula is still extraperitoneal the inflow is usually a drip unless the patient is very obese (Figure 3.5).

15. When fluid in, close roller on connecting tube and remove from cannula. Re-insert introducer to about 2 cm from tip of cannula. Slowly advance cannula aiming towards back of pelvis. Stop if there is resistance or pain (Figure A3.6).

16. When cannula judged to be at maximum possible depth withdraw introducer and reconnect connecting tube. Open rollers and observe drainage. The fluid should return as a continuous stream for most of the cycle. At least half the initial cycle must be returned reasonably quickly before the cannula can be judged satisfactory.

17. If fluid return poor, try withdrawing cannula 2 cm and observing effect. If return is still poor a flank approach may be necessary. Sometimes it is worth running in a further 500 to 1000 ml of dialysate. If all this is returned dialysis can be continued. Otherwise the cannula must be replaced at a fresh site.

18. When the cannula is working insert a purse string suture around. Do not pull so tight that skin necrosis will ensue. A snug watertight fit is all that is required. Leave ends of stitch long (Figure A3.7).

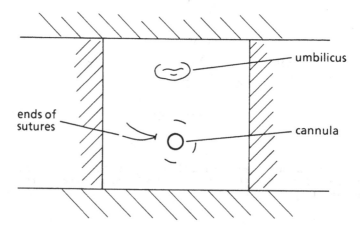

Figure A3.7 The position of the purse string suture around the cannula is shown

19.   Close roller on connecting tube and remove. Trim off excess cannula
       to 3 cm above the skin with sterile scissors or scalpel. Slip metal disc
       over cannula, slide down to just above skin and crimp onto cannula
       with fine artery forceps. Replace connecting tube (Figures A3.8 and
       A3.9).

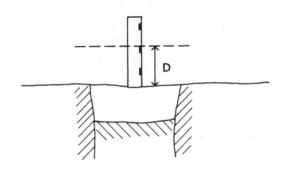

Figure A3.8 The cannula is trimmed approximately 3 cm (D) above the skin

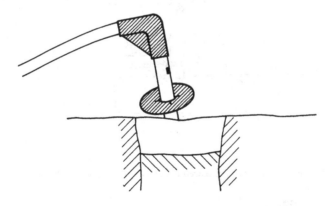

Figure A3.9 The metal disc is crimped on to the cannula just above the skin and the
connecting tube is re-attached

20.   Tie ends of suture around connecting tube. This reduces chances of
       pulling cannula out accidentally.
21.   Slip two folded small gauze swabs under metal disc to prevent it cutting
       into the skin. Place several swabs either side of cannula on top of disc.
       Cover whole of dressing with elastoplast (Figures A3.10 and A3.11).

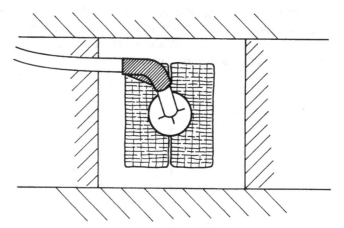

Figure A3.10 Two gauze swabs are folded underneath the metal disc and either side of the cannula

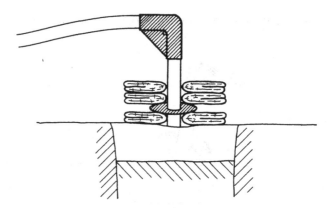

Figure A3.11 Further folded swabs are placed either side of the cannula above the disc

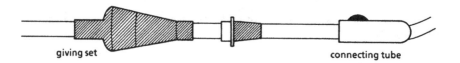

giving set   connecting tube

Figure A3.12 The junction between the giving set and the connecting tube must be taped to prevent accidental disconnection

22. Tape down connecting tube with elastoplast. This is most important as it avoids the tubing pulling directly on the cannula.

23. Tape junction of giving set and connecting tube to prevent disconnection (Figure A3.12).

24. Doctor to write prescription for exact regime, i.e. additives, cycle volume, type of fluid, dwell time, etc.

General comments

Normally a site should be chosen about 3 to 6 cm below the umbilicus. Avoid any obviously inflamed or infected areas. An alternative site is in the flank almost parallel to the umbilicus and outside the line drawn from the femoral artery at the groin to the umbilicus. This avoids damaging the inferior epigastric artery. If possible do not insert a cannula close to a scar or any abdominal opening (see sections on stoma, etc.). Try to make the length of the incision small enough so that the cannula dilates the hole making a watertight seal with the skin. Occasionally there is considerable resistance to advancing the cannula and the scalpel may have to be inserted up to the hilt to permit peritoneal entry.

For children a paediatric cannula is used. This has the same bore but the side holes extend only half as far up the cannula. It is wise to fill the abdomen with a fine needle prior to cannula insertion. See sections on choice of volume and dwell for details regarding peritoneal dialysis in children.

Removal of old cannula

1. Remove all tapes, plaster, etc. Gently remove all swabs.
2. Swab suture line and skin around cannula with povidone-iodine.
3. Pull gently on stitch with forceps and cut with stitch cutter. Remove stitch.
4. Gently withdraw cannula. Cut off tip with sterile scissors and place in sterile universal container for culture.
5. Clean skin again with povidone-iodine.
6. Apply dry dressing and tape.

If necessary, after step 5 doctor to infiltrate with local anaesthetic and insert a purse string suture. This must not be done if the site is obviously infected.

Trolley setting for cannula removal

Povidone-iodine
Stitch cutter
Small dressing pack
Sterile scissors
Sterile universal container
Tape

Cannula replacement **D**

The technique is similar to that for initial catheter insertion. Choose a different site. Even if the original hole appears clean it is wise to move a short distance, say about 2 cm. If the original hole is inflamed then the new cannula must be inserted well away, e.g. in the flank if the previous one was in the mid-line. Should the original cannula still be in place it can be used to fill the abdomen prior to insertion of the new one. Check the new catheter is functioning properly and then remove the old one. It is not necessary to routinely suture the original hole and this should certainly be avoided if it is inflamed. Normally a hole will close within hours if the abdomen is not distended by continuing dialysis. However, if the hole is clean and significant leakage occurs, a simple purse string silk suture will usually suffice. Whether or not a suture is used the original site requires cleaning with povidone-iodine and then a dry dressing. Should leakage occur despite these measures then try reducing the cycle volume by half or stop the dialysis for 24 hours. This is almost always sufficient to solve the problem.

Daily dressing technique for peritoneal dialysis cannula

Trolley requirements

Small dressing pack
Povidone-iodine solution
Hydrogen peroxide 3% (if needed)
Elastoplast strapping (new box)
Disposable dressing bag
Bag for reusable items

Procedure

1. Use aseptic technique and wear a mask.
2. Remove the old dressing without tugging at the cannula.
3. Swab the skin around the cannula with povidone-iodine solution, starting from the inside out.
4. If the cannula site is crusted use povidone-iodine or hydrogen peroxide 3% to soak off crusts.
5. Dry the site with the same procedure.
6. Ensure that the metal disc is not cutting into the abdomen by placing two small half folded swabs under the disc.
7. Place two half folded swabs either side of the cannula (folded edge nearest cannula), on top of the disc.
8. Cut two short lengths of clean elastoplast (from new box) and tape down the dressing above and below the cannula.
9. The connecting tube of the cannula should be strapped neatly to the abdomen with elastoplast to prevent the cannula from being tugged and disconnected from the giving set.
10. Ensure the junction of the giving set and connecting tube is securely taped to prevent disconnection.

Special nursing care of a patient having peritoneal dialysis

1. If the patient is in bed he must be sat upright or at least semi-recumbent as soon as possible.
2. As soon as his condition allows, he should be sat out of bed.
3. Request physiotherapy for chest and leg exercises.
4. Fluid intake to be prescribed by the doctor and a strict fluid balance chart kept.
5. 60 gram or more protein diet to be given at the doctor's discretion.
6. Accurate records of the dialysis should be kept and 24-hour totals of the recovered dialysate fluid made.
7. The patient should be weighed daily at the same time each day when abdomen is empty.
8. At least 4-hourly temperature, pulse and blood pressure should be recorded and charted.
9. Peritoneal dialysis pain can be relieved by adding lignocaine 1% 1 ml per litre, at the doctor's discretion.
10. Pain can be caused by allowing air to enter into the abdomen or by running a too hot or too cold dialysate fluid into the abdomen.
11. Sometimes a systemic analgesic or sedative may need to be given.

12.   If the peritoneal dialysis is running continuously, the cannula should not be spigotted off for any reason. The Y tape giving set should not be changed unless it becomes contaminated, blocked or there has been accidental contamination.

13.   When the peritoneal dialysis is running 12-hourly, ensure that patient is fully drained out. Close all roller clamps, assemble bags and lines as a neat package using elastic bands.

14.   Whenever the cannula is touched, e.g. during dressing or declotting, a trolley must be laid up and the procedure performed strictly aseptically.

15.   The bedside peritoneal dialysis tray must be relaid daily.

16.   Peritoneal dialysis specimens should not be collected from the drainage bag but from the rubber insert of the tubing set.

17.   Dressings of cannulae should be performed daily whether the patient is 'on' or 'off' dialysis (see procedure).

18.   Measuring cylinders to be cleaned daily with hypochlorite. Cylinders are also 'swilled' with Phenolic 2% (Stericol disinfectant) after every drainage.

19.   Daily trolley procedures:
   a) Trolley stripped, washed with detergent and hard surface cleaned with disinfectant such as chlorhexidine.
   b) Fresh incontinence pad used.
   c) Relaid with - Microtouch (non-sterile gloves)
                     - receiver with appropriate syringes and needles
                     - drugs as required
                     - alcoholic wipes for cleaning drug ampoules
                     - alcoholic chlorhexidine (Hibisol)
                     - 'sharps' box
                     - CAPD bag clamps soaking in alcoholic chlorhexidine

Bag change procedure

1.   When PD fluid has drained fully from the patient, close rollers on the tubing.

2.   Remove new bags from the heater (37 degrees C) and wash hands thoroughly.

3.   Clean top shelf of trolley with a hard surface disinfectant.

4. Open new bags if outer cover is intact and check six things:
    - Volume of bag
    - Concentration
    - Expiry date
    - Fluid is clear
    - Any leaks?
    - Sterile connection cover in place
5. Lay bags on clean surface of trolley.
6. Wash hands again.
7. Clean rubber injection ports on bags with alcohol swabs and leave to dry.
8. Clean rubber bung of multidose vial and/or break point of glass ampoule of any additives (e.g. heparin/antibiotics) with alcohol swab and leave to dry.
9. Draw up additives (in the case of glass ampoules dispose of any remaining drug).
10. Inject additives into both bags (dividing quantity between both bags).
11. Place bag clamp around both bag outlets, leaving sterile covers intact.
12. Lay old bags alongside new bags on the trolley.
13. Place bag clamps around each old bag outlet.
14. Rub hands with alcoholic chlorhexidine (Hibisol).
15. Remove sterile cover from empty port of new bag.
16. Remove spike from old bag and immediately insert into new bag avoiding any risk of contamination.
17. Repeat procedure for second bag.
18. Remove bag clamps, invert both bags to mix drugs.
19. Suspend new bags on drip stand and open rollers to commence flow.
20. Soak bag clamps in chlorhexidine between bag changes.
21. Discard old bags and remaining disposables.

Emptying of drainage bags

1. Put on plastic apron and disposable non-sterile gloves.
2. Ensure clamp is on drainage arm.
3. Empty bag contents into patient's own measuring cylinder.
4. Dip outlet as deep as possible into gallipot or universal container of povidone-iodine and then replace clamped off tube back into holder.
5. Measure fluid in cylinder.
6. Dispose of fluid down drain.
7. Swill cylinder with phenolic disinfectant 2% (Stericol)
8. Record outflow volume on dialysis chart.

Disconnection

1. Close rollers on connecting tube and giving set next to rubber injection sleeve. Remove tape from junction. Close all remaining rollers.
2. Wear mask, wash hands, put on sterile gloves.
3. Place sterile towel under connection. Scrub connection between giving set and connecting tube with swab soaked in povidone-iodine for 1 minute. Discard swab. Replace with fresh one soaked in iodine and leave wrapped around connection for 5 minutes.
4. Unwrap swab, take two sterile swabs, one in each hand, disconnect tubing set and place sterile rubber cap from Silastic catheter set over end of connecting tube.
5. Thoroughly dry cap and tube. Tape cap in position onto tube. Coil connecting tube on abdomen and tape down in comfortable position.
6. Discard whole of giving set, drainage bag, etc.

The rubber cap from a Silastic catheter set must be used. These caps can be purchased separately. A spigot is totally unsuitable.

Trolley setting for disconnection

Small dressing pack
1 packet of sterile gauze swabs
Povidone-iodine
Sterile gloves
Sterile rubber cap (suitable for Silastic catheter)

Reconnection

1. Prepare giving set. Put up fresh fluid with any necessary additives. Connect drainage bag. Run fluid through but leave sterile cover on patient end of tubing.
2. Remove strapping holding connecting tube to abdomen and straighten tube out. Remove any tape around rubber cap.
3. Mask, wash hands for 3 minutes, put on sterile gloves.
4. Place sterile towel under rubber cap.
5. Scrub around cap with swab soaked in povidone-iodine, for 1 minute. Discard swab. Place further iodine soaked swab around cap and leave for 5 minutes.

6. Undo swab. Gently slide off cap. Helper to pull off cover on end of tubing set and push into connecting tube without touching.
7. Open rollers and commence dialysis.
8. Dress cannula as described under daily dressing.
9. Place rubber cap in universal container nearly full of povidone-iodine. Caps can be re-used extensively.
10. Dry tubing. Retape connecting set to abdomen. Discard used swabs, etc.
11. *Tape junction of giving set and connecting tube* to prevent accidental disconnection.

Trolley setting for reconnection

Small dressing pack
Povidone-iodine
Sterile gloves
Tape

Bloodstained fluid   **D**

It is very common to have slightly bloodstained fluid after cannula insertion. This usually clears in a few cycles. Very occasionally bloodstaining may persist for some days. Heparin should be added to the fresh fluid at a concentration of 500 units per litre until the blood clears macroscopically to prevent clotting of the cannula. If haemorrhage is very severe check there is no obvious bleeding point at the entry site. Treat any shock with whole blood transfusion. If haemorrhage appears to be intra-abdominal, severe and not stopping, a laparotomy is necessary but this is a rare occurence. The main precaution is to avoid the inferior epigastric artery by sticking strictly to the mid-line or keeping well out to the flank almost parallel to the umbilicus. Patients with coagulation disorders should have their problems corrected just prior to cannula insertion.

Haematoma of abdominal wall   **D**

Very occasionally bleeding in the abdominal wall may occur. This is particularly likely to happen in the rectus abdominus muscle due to injury to the inferior epigastric artery. The problem can be largely avoided if the cannula is inserted strictly in the mid-line or well out in the flank. If the haematoma is mild then only simple analgesics are required. Rarely the clot may require evacuation with ligation of the bleeding point.

Perforated bladder   **D**

This problem can occur during cannula insertion. It usually becomes obvious as the patient suddenly passes a large volume of fluid which is strongly positive for glucose. Treatment involves removing the peritoneal cannula, inserting a bladder catheter for a few days on *continuous* closed drainage and re-inserting the peritoneal cannula at a different angle or site. The problem is unlikely to occur if the patient is made to empty the bladder prior to insertion. If the patient cannot micturate or is unconscious, a soft urinary catheter should be passed and then removed after the cannula is in position.

Perforated bowel   **D**

See section on faeculent fluid.

Pain in abdomen

Pain may occur soon after cannula insertion or if there is any peritonitis. Early pain often seems to be a jet effect, i.e. the fluid running in seems to hit some tender spot on the peritoneal surface. Prevention involves advancing the cannula slowly on insertion and stopping if any resistance occurs. This particular pain usually subsides within a few cycles but if it persists the effect of running in the fluid more slowly, i.e. as a fast drip, should be tried. If this does not relieve the problem after several cycles then the addition of 1-2 ml of 1% lignocaine to the bag prior to infusion may help.

Pain due to peritonitis may require oral or parenteral analgesics but will disappear once the inflammation subsides.

Another possible cause of pain is air bubbles in the fluid. If the level in the bubble trap is too low air will be swept into the abdomen. This may cause pain. The air will be absorbed fairly quickly if no more enters. Check the bubble trap and ensure it is at least half full. If air is the cause of pain then the symptom will disappear within a few hours of correction.

If the fluid is too hot then the patient will get quite severe pain. Check the bag temperature. It should be just warm to touch.

Fluid will not run in

Check that the rollers on the giving set are all open. Make sure there is no kink anywhere in the tubing between the fluid and the cannula. Ensure the giving set has been fully inserted into the bag. Sometimes repositioning the patient may relieve the problem. Very rarely an imperforate giving set is the cause, in which case change the tubing. Finally, try flushing the cannula using full aseptic techniques. If this fails to relieve the problem a new cannula may be necessary.

Fluid is slow running in

If the cannula and tubing are functioning normally then 2 litres of fluid should run into the abdomen in not much more than 15 minutes. If inflow is significantly slower then check the same points as in section on failure of fluid to run in.

However, a fault in the cannula is the most likely cause. It should be aseptically flushed and if necessary replaced.

Fluid will not run out

Check that all the rollers are open and that there is no kink in the tubing. Sometimes an air lock may impede flow. Ask the patient to cough or bear down. The increased intra-abdominal pressure will almost invariably overcome any air lock. Sometimes changing the patient's position may solve the problem. Occasionally constipation may impede drainage. The induction of a bowel action may well improve matters. If this fails the fault lies in the cannula and it will require to be flushed in an aseptic manner. Cannula replacement will be necessary if there is no response to these measures.

Fluid is slow to run out

From most adults 1-2 litre cycles will run out in 30 minutes if the system is working properly. If 2 litres are taking longer than 1 hour to run out then this is too slow. Furthermore, the fluid should run out as a constant stream until about three quarters or more of the cycle has been collected and only then slow down to a drip. If half the cycle or more comes out as a drip the system is not satisfactory. If more efficient dialysis or fluid removal is required then the same procedure as with total failure to run out should be followed. However, in some patients a decision may be made that the dialysis is temporarily adequate for that individual. In this situation a slow run out can to a certain extent mimic CAPD but the technical failure should not be forgotten as it is likely to get worse with adverse effects on the patient.

Flushing cannula

If poor flow appears to be due to a blocked cannula then flushing may solve the problem. This is particularly likely to be helpful if there is visible fibrin or clot in the tubing or drainage bag. Proceed as follows.

1.   Put on mask.
2.   Close rollers either side of junction between giving set and cannula connecting tube. Remove tape from junction.
3.   Wash hands.
4.   Open dressing pack. Pour povidone-iodine into gallipot. Drop on to sterile field a 20 ml syringe and a 21 gauge needle.
5.   Aseptically draw up 1000 units heparin. Sterilise injection port on a 250 ml bag of saline with alcohol wipe and inject heparin into bag.
6.   Wash hands and put on sterile gloves.
7.   Place sterile towel under tubing connection.
8.   Wrap povidone-iodine soaked swab around connection. Press firmly to ensure complete wetting. Leave for 5 minutes.
9.   Sterilise injection port on bag with alcohol wipe. Using syringe and needle draw up 10 ml of heparinised saline. Remove needle.
10. Disconnect giving set from connecting tube. Keep iodine swab around tubing end and lay so that it does not move on sterile towel.
11. Insert syringe into connecting tube (Figure A4). Open roller and aspirate.

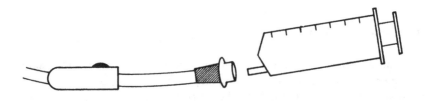

Figure A4 Flushing the cannula. The syringe should be inserted into the end of the connecting tube

24

12. If clots or fibrin appear close roller and discard syringe contents. Reaspirate until no further material comes free.
13. If no fluid can be obtained, try injecting syringe contents into cannula. Sometimes vigorous pushing and sucking will restore patency. Use fresh heparinised saline as necessary.
14. When there is free flow in and out of cannula close roller, discard syringe, wipe end of connecting tube with povidone-iodine and reinsert tubing.
15. Wipe off excess iodine with a dry sterile swab and then open rollers and recommence dialysis.

If free flow cannot be obtained then either replace cannula or consider urokinase. Cannulae tend to block from bleeding soon after insertion or if there is infection causing exudation. Always culture the fluid after dealing with a block and consider whether antibiotics are required. Heparin is also advisable for 24 hours to prevent fibrin plugging.

Trolley setting for flushing cannula

Small dressing pack
20 ml syringe
21 gauge needle
Heparin 1000 units/ml
250 ml saline bag (0.9% sodium chloride)
Povidone-iodine
Sterile gloves
Alcohol wipes

Use of urokinase

If a cannula cannot be freed with flushing it may sometimes be worthwhile attempting to clear it with urokinase. Make up 25,000 or 50,000 units of the drug in 2 ml of sterile saline. Aseptically disconnect the giving set from the connecting tube, as described under flushing cannula, and then inject the 2 ml down the connecting tube. Close the roller and either cap the tube with a rubber cap from a Silastic catheter set or reconnect the giving set. Wait for at least 2 hours. If dialysis is not required urgently then an overnight wait is often worthwhile. Subsequently flush the cannula as previously described. If it is still not patent it is wiser to replace the cannula at a separate site than attempting to use more urokinase.

If there is a total blockage preventing the urokinase from being injected then aspirate the connecting tube with another syringe. Clamp the tube as close to the syringe as possible while maintaining suction. Remove the empty syringe and insert the syringe containing the urokinase into the connecting tube. Release the clamp and the previously created vacuum will suck in the drug allowing it to reach the site of obstruction. Continue as above.

When to sample

It is not necessary to sample PD fluid daily. In general if the outflow (effluent) is clear and the patient is asymptomatic then it is highly unlikely there is any peritoneal infection. The only exception to this rule occurs if the patient 's white blood cell count is very low. In this situation a daily sample is necessary until the count is back to normal.

A sample must be taken if the fluid is cloudy or if the patient has abdominal pain and/or a raised temperature. Samples should also be taken if there is fibrin visible even if the fluid appears to be clear or if contamination could have occurred. Bloodstained effluent requires culturing though usually proves sterile.

Sampling of fluid

When necessary a sample of the outflow should be obtained for culture. It is not possible to sample the drainage bag in a simple safe manner. The dialysis tubing set contains a rubber injection port or sleeve just prior to the connection with the cannula connection tube (Figure A5). This should be used for sampling as follows:

1. Assemble syringe and needle.
2. Wash hands. Put on non-sterile gloves. Wash gloved hands with alcoholic chlorhexidine (Hibisol).
3. Allow first 100 ml outflow to drain.
4. Close roller clamp between rubber and Y junction.
5. Clean rubber port with alcohol wipe. Allow alcohol to dry.
6. Aspirate 20 ml of fluid and transfer to sterile universal container. Aspirate further 10 ml of fluid and divide between standard aerobic and anaerobic blood culture bottles.
    Despatch to laboratory with request form.
7. Open clamp and allow outflow to continue.

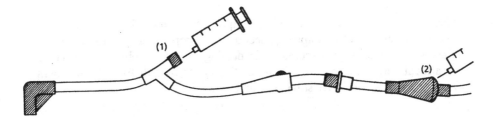

Figure A5 Samples for culture can be taken from the rubber injection port of the connecting tube (1). Alternatively they may be obtained from the rubber bulb on the patient end of the giving set (2).

Crusting around cannula

Slight crusting may occur and is not serious. Excessive crusting implies infection is present. The daily dressing of the exit site should include soaking any crust with povidone-iodine or hydrogen peroxide and then gentle removal with swabs. Do not pull if it will not come easily.

Redness around cannula

Minimal redness is acceptable but if the area affected spreads then infection is present. Neither local measures nor systemic antibiotics are likely to help. Cannula removal is necessary to solve the problem.

Infection around cannula   **D**

The signs of infection are initially redness with perhaps crust formation. Later actual skin ulceration with beads of pus are seen. Neither local measures nor systemic antibiotics will do more than temporarily damp things down. The correct procedure is to remove the cannula and, if necessary, replace at a different site. If there was only redness antibiotics are not essential. However, visible pus warrants an antibacterial agent. The commonest causative organism is a *Staphylococcus* and, therefore, a drug such as cloxacillin is appropriate until the results of a swab are available.

Leakage from old site

Usually the abdominal wall seals promptly after removal of a cannula. If leakage occurs then the simplest procedure is to stop the dialysis for 24 hours. This is almost invariably successful in dealing with the problem. Alternative treatments are reducing the volume of the cycles by half for 6 to 12 hours and/or trying an occlusive stitch around the hole.

Leakage around cannula   D

If the fluid leaks around the cannula there is a serious risk of infection. Check if the skin exit is clean. If it is, try a new purse-string suture and/or reduce volume of cycles by half. Should these measures fail to correct the problem within a few hours or the exit site is inflamed or crusted, then remove the cannula and re-insert at a new site if more dialysis is necessary. Usually the old exit seals quickly but may need an occluding stitch.

Leakage from tubing or cannula

Neither the tubing nor the cannula is self-sealing except for the rubber injection sleeve. If a leak occurs the relevant part must be replaced promptly. Do not attempt to seal with waterproof plaster, plastic spray, etc.

Cannula disappears   D

Rarely the cannula may disappear into the abdomen. This complication is made less likely if the metal disc is crimped firmly onto the cannula at the initial insertion. Unless infection is present the presence of the cannula in the peritoneal cavity causes very little trouble. A laparotomy is necessary to remove the cannula but this can be done when the patient has recovered. If infection is present then the cannula should be retrieved urgently. It is uncertain whether laparoscopic removal is feasible. Unfortunately the temporary cannula is not sufficiently radio-opaque for plain abdominal X-rays to be helpful.

Cannula moves out

Sometimes a peritoneal cannula may move so that there is more protruding from the abdomen. Do not push it back in as this will introduce infection. Instead, if there is a significant movement, e.g. one inch or more and the dialysis is still working satisfactorily, soak the exposed portion with povidone-iodine for at least 5 minutes, then trim to one inch above the skin with sterile scissors and replace the connecting arm immediately. Finally replace the padding around the cannula and retape as noted in the section on cannula insertion. If the dialysis is not working well replace the cannula at a new site. This must also be done if the exit site is inflamed or obviously infected.

Cloudy fluid   D

Cloudy fluid almost invariably means there are excess white cells, mainly polymorphs, present. The implication is that inflammation, i.e. peritonitis, is present. Though chemical irritation is possible as a cause, the vast majority of patients will prove to have a bacterial infection. A decision should be made whether to stop the peritoneal dialysis in which case the cannula *must* be removed. Usually the infection will then clear up spontaneously irrespective of whether antibiotics are given if there is no underlying bowel problem. Should a bowel disorder such as diverticulitis be present it must be treated medically or surgically on its own merits. Sometimes haemodialysis can be used as a temporary measure while the abdomen settles for 3-4 weeks.

If peritoneal dialysis is to be continued an appropriate antibiotic should be added to the fluid prior to infusion (see table of antibiotic doses pp. 30-31) and continued for up to a week after the fluid is clear and the cultures negative. If there is fibrin visible in the returned fluid heparin should be added to the inflow at a concentration of 500 units/litre to prevent the cannula getting blocked. Should the fluid not clear within 7 days then the cannula itself may well be acting as the focus of infection and should be removed. A new cannula in a new position may be tried but if the infection does not rapidly clear using the right antibiotic then peritoneal dialysis should be stopped, the cannula removed and haemodialysis used for up to 4 weeks as necessary before any attempt should be made to restart peritoneal dialysis.

Peritonitis   D

The signs of peritonitis are cloudy fluid, abdominal pain, tenderness and temperature. Cloudy fluid is often the first sign without any symptoms being present. If peritonitis is suspected then send fluid immediately for Gram stain and culture. On the basis of the Gram stain choose an appropriate antibiotic. Decide if dialysis is to continue. If not then remove cannula and treat with a systemic antibiotic. If dialysis is continuing then inspect the exit site. Should this be clean then add antibiotics to the fluid. Suggested doses of antibiotics are given in the table below. If the exit site is inflamed then take a swab for culture and replace the cannula at a fresh site, adding antibiotics to the fluid as before. A further guide to appropriate treatment may be given by checking all previous fluid cultures. Sometimes an organism is grown before there is much evidence of clinical peritonitis.

Many infections are controlled within 48 hours of starting drugs. A good guide to progress is the clearing of the fluid. Sometimes obvious strands of fibrin are seen. Heparin should then be added at a concentration of 500 units per litre until the fluid is no longer cloudy. Antibiotics should be continued for several days after the fluid is sterile but no trial of different times is available. The author's advice is 5-7 days after the fluid is clear. If the patient is sytemically ill then antibiotics should also be given parenterally but where infection appears to be local without much pain or temperature then antibiotics can be inserted in the fluid alone. There is little doubt that this usage is as effective, if not more effective, than parenteral antibiotics on their own.

If the infection is not under control within a week despite using the right antibiotic then the cannula must be removed as it has probably become colonised. A new one can be inserted but if there is not rapid clearing of the fluid the patient should be transferred to haemodialysis, all foreign bodies removed from the abdomen and antibiotics then given systemically.

Antibiotic dosage in PD fluid   D

Drug	Dosage
Amikacin	20 mg/litre
Gentamicin	8 mg/litre
Netilmicin	10 mg/litre
Tobramycin	8 mg/litre
Vancomycin	25 mg/litre
Cefotaxime	250 mg/litre
Cefuroxime	250 mg/litre
Ampicillin	125 mg/litre

Azlocillin	500 mg/litre
Cloxacillin	250 mg/litre
Mezlocillin	500 mg/litre
Piperacillin	200 mg/litre
Fusidic acid	50 mg/litre
Amphotericin B	5 mg/litre

N.B. Aminoglycosides and penicillins are probably incompatible in PD fluid at these concentrations. Cephalosporins may be mixed in the same bag as aminoglycosides but not the same syringe. All these antibiotics are compatible with heparin and potassium chloride in PD fluid. It is unwise to use fusidic acid on its own as resistance may develop rapidly. The use of the newer antibiotics such as aztreonam and ciprofloxacin for treating infections during intermittent peritoneal dialysis has not yet been reported. If necessary doses similar to those used in CAPD should be tried.

Notes on intraperitoneal aminoglycosides   **D**

Determining serum levels is most important.

Absorption across the peritoneum is usually in the range of 25-67% and, therefore, quite variable levels will be seen in different patients.

In renal patients being treated intraperitoneally with aminoglycosides the usual peak/trough pharmacokinetic profile does not occur. Instead an approximately constant serum level occurs which rises very gradually with time. The toxic serum level in these patients is determined by calculating that steady state level which produces an area under the elimination curve which is equal to that of the peak/trough curve. These levels are as shown below, and should not be exceeded.

	Normal parenteral usage			*Intraperitoneal usage*
Drug	*Peak*	*Trough*	*Frequency*	*Steady state 'toxic level'*
Amikacin	25 mg/l	9 mg/l	BD	16 mg/l
Gentamicin	8 mg/l	2 mg/l	TDS	4.5 mg/l
Netilmycin	16 mg/l	4 mg/l	BD	8.5 mg/l
Tobramycin	8 mg/l	2 mg/l	TDS	4.5 mg/l

If a steady state level much lower than that shown is found, the dosage may be increased if required. Indeed, increasing the dose in that instance may well be desirable since this will increase the concentration to which the bacteria are exposed; given that 'peak' concentrations are not achieved in these patients their infection may well not respond at low steady state levels.

If the steady state level exceeds that shown the dosage should obviously be reduced. It may be necessary to stop the aminoglycoside altogether for a short time.

Prophylactic antibiotics D

Antibiotics should not be given prophylactically without reason. However, if a contamination accident occurs such as a disconnection, then a 3 day course of intraperitoneal antibiotics using standard doses should be prescribed.

Faeculent fluid D

If the fluid is faeculent it will be a yellow-brown colour and smell of faeces. Should this be discovered it means there has been a bowel perforation. A further sign of bowel perforation due to the cannula is the sudden onset of watery diarrhoea positive for glucose. Usually this problem arises immediately after cannula insertion, i.e. the cannula pierced the bowel during the procedure. Perforation is more likely if ileus or intestinal obstruction is present or there are adhesions. Great care should be taken in starting peritoneal dialysis in an abdomen with any of these condition present. Bowel perforation is less likely to occur if the cannula is not advanced until the abdomen has been filled with fluid and then inserted gently, stopping if there is any resistance. If faeculent fluid occurs the cannula should be removed and a new one inserted at a different site. If peritoneal dialysis can be established then sometimes the perforation will seal rapidly. The patient should be given the standard treatment of nasogastric suction and i.v. fluid together with broad spectrum antibiotics including a drug to cover anaerobes. Patients should be closely observed and if there is any deterioration a laparotomy should be performed urgently. It may be possible to re-establish peritoneal dialysis at the close of the operation, the surgeon placing the cannula in the pelvis under direct vision. In this case it is probably advisable to change to a Tenckhoff type Silastic catheter. Postoperatively the fluid should contain heparin and an appropriate antibiotic. Fluid volumes should be kept low to avoid leakage, e.g. if 2 litres would be used normally use 500 ml cycles for a few days then slowly increase if no problem arises.

Erosion of bowel by a cannula which has been present for some time rarely, if ever, occurs. Faeculent fluid occurring some days after insertion probably means a spontaneous perforation due to some intrinsic bowel disease. In this case urgent laparotomy is required.

Multiple organisms   D

Most peritoneal infections are with a single organism. If the culture reports several bacteria then suspect that the sample was contaminated after leaving the patient. However, if the peritonitis is actually due to a bowel problem such as diverticulitis then multiple organisms may be grown. Usually a significant infection is accompanied by polymorphs. If the patient is well with no abnormal signs and the fluid draining is clear, then it is unlikely the organisms were actually present in the patient.

False positive cultures

If a patient has evidence of infection, particularly cloudy fluid, then any organism grown is almost certainly relevant. However, sometimes cultures may be falsely positive. A significant infection is usually accompanied by large numbers of white cells and all bacteriological reports should comment on the cell content of the spun deposit. Should the patient appear well, the fluid is clear and no or only a few white cells were seen, then the culture is probably falsely positive. One cause is taking the sample from the fluid after it has been placed in an open drainage cylinder. If any sample grows an organism, a further specimen should be obtained to confirm the diagnosis. Commonly a false positive culture is followed by a negative one. See section on sampling.

Fluid balance assessment   D

There is only one certain way of assessing the patient's fluid balance, namely daily weighing, if necessary using a bed weigher. However, it is helpful to have an ongoing idea of fluid removal during dialysis. The widely used 1 litre peritoneal dialysis bags in fact contain a minimum of 1 litre, usually with about 50 ml excess. This means that a more accurate fluid balance in respect of the dialysate is obtained if a 2 litre cycle is assumed to be 2100 ml. The drainage bag contains graduated markings but these are not very accurate, tending to over-read below 1 litre. It is essential to drain the completed outflow into a measuring cylinder to get the true volume returned.

When dialysing small children it is usual to dispense the fluid from a graduated drip chamber, e.g. Buretrol, and thus a very accurate measurement of fluid given in each cycle is obtained.

Fluid removal   **D**

The osmolality of the 1.36% dextrose fluid is similar to that of plasma from a severely uraemic patient. If fluid removal is required during the initial phase of treatment it is therefore necessary to use a more hypertonic solution. Should the patient be severely fluid overloaded and in particular have pulmonary oedema then all 3.86% dextrose is required. If this does not cause a significant excess outflow volume compared to inflow then a *few* bags of 6.36% dextrose can be used. When fluid removal is less urgent it is wiser to reduce the dialysis cycles to alternating 1.36% and 3.86%. If 2 litre cycles are used then 1 litre bags of each can be given as a mixture. This slows down the rate of fluid removal and lessens the chance of dehydration. Smaller volumes can also be mixed using a burette system for each bag. Once uraemia is well controlled even 1.36% dextrose fluid may have a significantly higher osmolality than the patient's plasma and fluid removal will continue. This is particularly likely to occur with smaller patients. A careful check on the total daily excess removed should be made as well as the patient's weight to ensure dehydration does not occur.

Failure to remove excess fluid   **D**

Sometimes, despite using hypertonic cycles, no extra fluid is removed. One cause may be a faulty cannula position. If the fluid is clear change the cannula to a new site trying to ensure as low an intrapelvic position but stopping if any resistance is felt. It is common experience that fluid removal often decreases when peritonitis occurs. If the fluid is cloudy suspect peritonitis and treat appropriately after sampling. When the inflammation subsides then the problem will resolve. If, however, the patient requires urgent fluid removal, whatever the cause, consider using ultrafiltration with a haemodialysis system.

Oedema of abdominal skin   **D**

This may be due to general fluid retention caused by renal failure in which case it will be evident on initial examination prior to cannula insertion. It will disappear if the dialysis is effective in removing fluid.

Another possibility is tracking of the dialysis fluid into the abdominal wall. This is most likely to occur if the cannula is not advanced sufficiently to place all the side holes in an intraperitoneal position. This type of oedema will only occur after dialysis has been running some hours or days and tends to slowly worsen. Replacing the cannula in a new position with more fluid removal will resolve the problem.

Oedema of genitalia   D

This has the same causes and requires the same management as oedema of the abdominal skin. Very occasionally it may be caused by fluid retention due to repeatedly 'losing' dialysis fluid intraperitoneally, i.e. the amount drained out is persistently less than that run in. If this appears to be happening try hypertonic cycles and if these fail replace the cannula. If fluid removal does not improve consider ultrafiltration using a haemodialysis system.

An unusual cause of genital oedema is the presence of an inguinal hernia sometimes previously unrecognised. A herniorrhaphy will be necessary to cure the problem.

Rarely localised swelling of the scrotum or labia is due to an open processus vaginalis so that the fluid flows directly from the peritoneal cavity into the genitalia. If this appears to be the cause then surgical repair is the only solution.

Dehydration   D

It is possible to remove too much fluid from a patient producing dehydration. The usual clinical signs of dry skin, sunken eyeballs, etc. will be present but this diagnosis is most often made because the patient becomes hypotensive in the absence of some other cause. It is more likely if hypertonic fluid is used but even 1.36% dextrose solution may on occasions remove a considerable amount of extra water, particularly from female patients. The treatment is to stop the dialysis if possible and rehydrate orally or intravenously depending on the severity of the clinical situation. Prevention requires attention to the daily weight and regard to the PD chart. If the weight is falling and no oedema is present, dehydration may be occurring. If the PD is removing large volumes of fluid ensure that overall water balance is maintained.

Hypotension   D

Hypotension may be a symptom of dehydration (see this section). It may also occur if bacteraemia occurs from peritonitis. Other causes will not be directly related to the dialysis. However, remember that uraemic patients may develop pericarditis with tamponade causing low blood pressure. If hypotension occurs stop the dialysis and treat the cause appropriately. Should peritonitis appear to be the problem either remove the cannula or recommence dialysis with added antibiotics. It is wise in this case to reduce the cycle volume until blood pressure improves. If hypotension is very severe, e.g. less than 80 mm Hg systolic in adults, it may not be possible to do a peritoneal dialysis as the presence of abdominal fluid may exacerbate the circulatory state. Dialysis should be postponed until the situation has improved. Do not forget that in a uraemic patient as fluid is removed the need for hypotensive drugs usually decreases otherwise marked hypotension may occur.

Hypertension   D

Hypertension does not commonly occur as a consequence of peritoneal dialysis unless there is a failure of fluid removal when fluid overload may cause a raised blood pressure. Pain and discomfort from the procedure may contribute to hypertension. If a patient requires peritoneal dialysis the blood pressure will almost always fall if sufficient fluid is removed. In fact, the failure to control hypertension is usually a sign of continuing fluid overload. Hypotensive drugs may need to be given in the interim particularly if there are hypertensive complications present.

Ascites   D

The presence of ascites prior to commencing dialysis should raise the possibility of liver disease. If the ascites is purely part of a general fluid overload then dialysis is in fact easier as the intra-abdominal fluid reduces the chance of any organ perforation. However, if the ascites is secondary to liver disease and/or portal hypertension, then it will contain considerable amounts of protein. Draining this fluid off and using peritoneal dialysis will cause extensive protein depletion and could well lead to the patient's death. Do not perform peritoneal dialysis in this clinical situation.

Ascites due to metastatic carcinoma would not normally warrant any dialysis irrespective of the presence of renal failure.

Should any ascitic fluid be present at the start of dialysis it must be cultured for ordinary pathogens and also tuberculosis since tuberculous peritonitis can occur in uraemic patients.

If fluid accumulation following cessation of dialysis occurs, it may well be due to fluid overload. Once again a sample of fluid should be obtained to exclude infection including tuberculosis.

Hypoalbuminaemia   D

There is an inevitable protein loss with peritoneal dialysis. The less dialysis, the less the loss. Hence losses are not so great with CAPD as with continuous flushing cycles. It is essential that the patient's protein intake be increased if he/she has peritoneal dialysis, e.g. should they have been given 40 gram/day then this must be increased to at least 60 gram/day while they have dialysis. If patients eat well then the serum albumin will stay normal or fall slightly but usually not below 30 gram/litre. However, infection causes a considerable increase in protein loss and the serum albumin will inevitably fall, sometimes to very low levels. Once infection is controlled then excess loss stops and the serum albumin will rise. Sometimes it is necessary to give oral protein supplements or protein infusions but this will depend on the individual patient's clinical state and no general guidance can be given.

Obesity   D

It is perfectly feasible to perform peritoneal dialysis on these patients. However, extreme obesity (>100 kg) may cause problems. The major difficulty is getting sufficient cannula into the peritoneal cavity. Some of the side holes may be above the peritoneal membrane and oedema of the abdominal wall will ensue. Another problem occurs in those with a large apron of fat. The cannula may go in all right but when the patient sits or stands the apron 'flows' down and the cannula rolls so that it is pointing upwards instead of down to the pelvis. Sometimes a flank approach will overcome this problem as there is less movement. If difficulties occur the patient should be transferred to haemodialysis. It is feasible to insert a Silastic catheter via a laparotomy and ensure its pelvic position but this is a high risk procedure in a patient with extreme obesity and renal failure.

Dialysis after laparotomy

This is a common problem. If the operation was done more than 48 hours prior to requiring dialysis and there are no drains, stomata, etc. then peritoneal dialysis can be started with little difficulty. The cannula should be inserted the opposite side of the abdomen to the laparotomy wound. Be careful if ileus is still present. If drains or stomata are present then extra care is required (see relevant sections). Sometimes dialysis is necessary soon after a laparotomy. This means the patient will probably still have an ileus and there is also a risk of wound leakage. The latter problem is less likely if small volumes of fluid are used, e.g. 500 ml for an average sized adult, and the cycle size slowly increased over a few days. Avoidance of dwell will also reduce the chances of leakage.

However it is safer to use haemodialysis rather than risk the dangers of inserting a rigid cannula. If dialysis is likely to be necessary very soon after a laparotomy and peritoneal dialysis is preferred then it is better to ask the surgeon to implant a Silastic peritoneal catheter at the close of the operation. This avoids the risk of bowel perforation and at least initially ensures the catheter is in the pelvis. Silastic cannulae must be flushed with heparinised dialysate as soon as the patient leaves theatre to prevent obstruction by fibrin. Usually 500 ml flushing cycles will be adequate for most adults. Should wound leakage occur then the cycle volume should be halved or the dialysis stopped for 12 hours. Persistent leakage means haemodialysis should be used instead.

Ileus, obstruction, adhesions   D

If any of these are present then there is a higher risk of bowel perforation or difficulty in obtaining a good return of the fluid. Cannulae should only be inserted into such patients by those with considerable experience of peritoneal dialysis. It is vital the abdomen is filled with fluid before the cannula is advanced. Stop if there is significant resistance. Try and avoid a site close to laparotomy scars to lessen the risk of hitting any bowel stuck under the wound. If difficulties occur consider changing to haemodialysis.

Colostomy, ileostomy, ureterostomy, conduit   D

The presence of any of these stomata makes peritoneal dialysis potentially more difficult. However, a successful dialysis can sometimes be established. In general the cannula should be inserted the opposite side of the abdomen to the stoma. If the patient has only had one or two laparotomies then it is unlikely there will be many adhesions. On the other hand multiple scars imply a much higher risk and haemodialysis should be considered. The presence of a stoma increases the risk of infection. It is important to maintain a water-tight seal around the orifice to prevent the excretions reaching the cannula site. In addition the cannula site dressings must be changed daily and more frequently if there is any suspicion of contamination. Repeated contamination means the patient should be switched to haemodialysis or infection will be inevitable.

Abdominal fistulae and drains   D

Fistulae and drains make peritoneal dialysis an unsatisfactory and potentially dangerous procedure. There are bound to be some adhesions particularly with fistulae. Dialysis can sometimes be started but often the fluid will return via the drain hole. This greatly increases the risk of infection and may make dialysis less efficient as the fluid probably flows in a narrow tract to the drain site instead of diffusing widely. Haemodialysis should seriously be considered if there is significant return of fluid via fistulae, etc. If peritoneal dialysis must be continued an attempt should be made to collect the fluid in a sterile closed system. If dialysate pours straight out of a drain as soon as it runs in the cannula, then clamping the drain may work. However, peritoneal dialysis should be abandoned as soon as possible or peritonitis is highly likely.

Blood urea does not fall   D

In the majority of patients a well-working peritoneal dialysis will control uraemia easily. It is not uncommon for the blood urea to change very little in the first 12 hours of dialysis and then to fall slowly. However, occasionally the blood urea fails to fall and may continue to rise. Check the dialysis is working properly with a reasonable number of cycles being performed. Make sure the patient is having adequate calories to reduce protein catabolism. If the uraemia does not improve the patient is probably hypercatabolic and requires haemodialysis instead.

Disequilibrium   D

Dialysis disequilibrium with confusion, coma and fits was originally described following rapid treatment of uraemia by haemodialysis. Whereas the full blown picture does not occur with peritoneal dialysis there are occasional patients who remain or become semi-conscious for some days following the start of treatment. Subsequently they spontaneously get better with no sequelae. Other causes of altered consciousness should be looked for but if by exclusion the condition appears to be related to the uraemia, the only treatment necessary is to control the renal failure by dialysis as necessary. Altered consciousness due to uraemia or disequilibrium should not persist more than a week if the renal failure is treated.

Hyperkalaemia   D

Peritoneal dialysis is usually very efficient at controlling a raised serum potassium. If the serum potassium does not fall check the dialysis is running well and being performed correctly. Ensure no potassium-containing drugs are being given and that there is no potassium being added to the PD fluid. Check that the diet or drinks do not contain excess potassium. If the problem persists then haemodialysis should be considered urgently.

Hypokalaemia   D

Though peritoneal dialysis fluid containing potassium is available, most units start treatment with a potassium-free fluid as hyperkalaemia is a common indication for treatment. However, hypokalaemia can easily be produced. The electrolytes must be checked at least daily once dialysis has commenced and if the plasma potassium is falling then potassium chloride should be added to the fluid. The usual dose is 0.25 g/l which is equivalent to about 3.2 mmol/l. Occasionally hypokalaemia occurs because the patient is taking a low potassium diet as well as being dialysed. Sometimes when large doses of frusemide are used for uraemic patients, hypokalaemia may ensue.

Hyperglycaemia   D

All commercially available peritoneal dialysis fluid contains glucose. Most non-diabetic patients will not have significant hyperglycaemia despite the absorption of glucose from the peritoneal cavity. Sustained use of 6.36% dextrose containing fluid can, however, produce a grossly raised blood sugar to more than 50 mmol/l (900 mg%). For this reason this particular fluid should only be used for one or two cycles at the most. Diabetic patients will rapidly become hyperglycaemic when treated by peritoneal dialysis and require extra insulin. Those who previously required a diet alone or oral hypoglycaemic drugs may well have to switch to insulin. Occasional patients who probably had sub-clinical glucose intolerance prior to the procedure become frankly diabetic with peritoneal dialysis. Since during intermittent peritoneal dialysis the patient is not always in a clinically stable situation it is wiser to give the insulin parenterally and not intraperitoneally (see use of insulin in Silastic cannula section).

Hypercalcaemia   D

Very occasionally patients may have renal failure and severe hypercalcaemia, e.g. myeloma. Most commercial dialysis fluids contain calcium. However, a large hospital pharmacy which manufactures sterile fluids can make a special batch of low or zero calcium dialysate. If such can be obtained then peritoneal dialysis with this fluid will cause a rapid reduction in serum calcium which will improve the patient and may help renal function.

Manufacturers will produce low calcium dialysate to order but may not always have it in stock.

Chest complications   D

All patients with uraemia are more prone to infection than normal individuals and sepsis is the single most important cause of death in acute renal failure. Peritoneal dialysis can cause pulmonary problems. Patients on continuous dialysis are likely to get basal atelectasis with superimposed infection. Occasionally pleural effusions may occur. Patients who have pre-existing lung or heart problems may find peritoneal dialysis causes respiratory embarrassment. If there is diaphragmatic irritation such as by peritonitis then shoulder tip pain may occur. To reduce the chances of lung problems dialysis should be cut to 12 hours a day as soon as possible. Physiotherapy should be given and the patients got out of bed as much as possible as well as being encouraged to cough. If respiratory embarrassment occurs then reduce the cycle volume by half.

Very occasionally patients may develop a massive pleural effusion due to the dialysis fluid passing through a foramen in the diaphragm. If this occurs the glucose content of the pleural fluid will be many times higher than that of the blood. Should this happen peritoneal dialysis will have to be discontinued and haemodialysis considered.

Air under diaphragm   D

Erect films of the abdomen commonly show air under the diaphragm in patients on peritoneal dialysis. This is of no serious significance, though may cause pain (see section on pain). The only problem that could arise is if such a patient were to be suspected of having a perforation of the stomach or bowel. In this situation the presence of air under diaphragm could not be used to confirm the diagnosis and other investigations would be necessary.

Hernia   D

Intermittent peritoneal dialysis performed as a temporary measure does not have a high chance of causing a hernia (see Silastic catheter section). However, any pre-existing abdominal hernia will be exacerbated and will become very difficult to reduce while fluid is in the abdomen because of increased intra-abdominal pressure. The presence of any hernia should be noted and the possibility of strangulation considered if peritonitis occurs.

Choice of cycle volume   D

In general most adults (> 50 kg) will tolerate a 2 litre cycle volume without much discomfort. Patients of 30 to 40 kg will require a 1 litre cycle. Those between 40 and 50 kg will vary in their tolerance and the volume must be assessed on the basis of patient comfort and the efficiency of dialysis.

Children require a cycle volume of 30 ml/kg. This is conveniently dispensed via a graduated drip chamber, e.g. Buretrol.

Dwell times   D

The longer the fluid stays in the abdomen the more the concentration of urea, etc. in the dialysate will approach that of blood. However, long dwell times mean less cycles and in acutely ill patients possibly less total removal of uraemic metabolites. Most of the excess fluid removed by osmosis is intraperitoneal in about 30 minutes. Studies have shown that leaving the fluid for 15 minutes shut off in the abdomen gives as good results in-terms of fall in blood urea as letting it run straight out after inflow. The actual practice adopted will depend on the patient's needs and the staffing situation. Small children should have a dwell time of 15 to 30 minutes as otherwise the whole cycle may only take 10 minutes and hardly any exchange will take place. For adults if the unit is short-staffed it may well be better to start outflow immediately after inflow as otherwise the dialysis may be forgotten and very few cycles will be performed. If a patient can be specialled by one nurse then a 15 minute dwell should be tried. However, if outflow is rather slow so that a 2 litre cycle is taking an hour or more to complete, the patient is effectively having a dwell so no extra is required.

Continuous or intermittent dialysis   D

When patients are first started on peritoneal dialysis they will usually need treatment continuously for 24 to 48 hours. Once they are better dialysis should be reduced to 12 hours a day or less if clinical circumstances allow. This reduction will help to prevent pulmonary complications and allow the patient to be kept more mobile. There will be some patients, however, who will need continuous dialysis because of catabolism or the fluid load inherent in maintaining nutrition.

Choice of fluid   D

There are a number of different fluid compositions available as well as different bag sizes. The section on fluid volumes gives guidelines on optimum cycle amounts dependent on the patient's size. Besides the standard 1 litre containers, bags for use with a CAPD system are available in 300 ml, 500 ml, 1000 ml, 1500 ml and 2000 ml amounts and these can be used for ordinary peritoneal dialysis. Ten litre cans and 5 litre bags are marketed for use with automatic machines.

Currently in the United Kingdom dextrose concentrations of 1.36%, 2.27%, 3.86% and 6.36% are available. The section on fluid removal comments on their usage. In other parts of the world the dextrose concentrations may be expressed as the hydrated compound (the United Kingdom bags are expressed as anhydrous dextrose) giving percentages of 1.5% and 4.25% (instead of 1.36% and 3.86%).

The dialysate will usually contain acetate or lactate though the latter is preferred (see Section B, Peritoneal sclerosis). These are incorporated to back-diffuse into the body and then be metabolised to bicarbonate thus buffering uraemic acidosis. Bicarbonate containing peritoneal dialysis fluid is technically difficult to produce.

The usual sodium concentration of dialysate is about 140 mmol/l. A low sodium dialysate (130 mmol/l) is available. Some patients, particularly those who have a lot of fluid removal during peritoneal dialysis, may develop hypernatraemia as the ultrafiltrate itself is low in sodium. It is claimed that dialysis against a low sodium dialysate prevents hypernatraemia without causing hyponatraemia.

The most widely used peritoneal dialysis fluids contain no potassium. It is, therefore, incumbent upon the clinician to prescribe any potassium additives as necessary for the individual patient. There are now available some CAPD type bags with potassium already added by the manufacturer. For acutely ill patients it is better to prescribe individually. For long-term patients such as those having CAPD it would be logical to treat persisting hypokalaemia with dialysis fluid containing potassium added prior to sterilisation. This might reduce the need for oral potassium supplements and avoid the risk of infection inherent in adding potassium to the bags at the bedside.

It should be noted that not every possible combination of these different constituents of the fluid is currently available.

The doctor should prescribe the fluid appropriate for each individual patient.

Heating of fluid D

It is possible to use fluid at room temperature but this can be uncomfortable for some patients. In small sick children there would be a slight risk of hypothermia. Bags of fluid should be heated by dry heat preferably in a thermostatically controlled incubator to 38 degrees C. A laboratory type incubator with a back-up overheat cut-off and alarm has proved very satisfactory. A towel-covered radiator will suffice in emergency. There are available various pieces of equipment to help with heating. Messrs Vickers market an in-line heater but this requires additional special tubing. There are flat plate heaters originally designed for CAPD bags at home but these only heat one or two bags at a time. Microwave ovens are not recommended as bags of fluid have ruptured due to local overheating. The various semi-automatic PD machines often include a heating system but extra tubing is required. Bags should only be warm to touch and not hot or the patient will get severe pain.

Peritoneal dialysis machines D

The peritoneal dialysis system can be automated to varying degrees. The simplest machine consists of a timer-controlled clamping device controlling inflow and outflow. More sophisticated equipment uses pre-sterilised fluid in 5 or 10 litre containers and after heating controls volume and time of inflow, dwell and outflow. Reversed osmosis machines purify water by reversed osmosis and filtration and then mix the product with sterile concentrate. The machines then control the dialysis cycle via timers.

Usage of these types of equipment reduces nursing work as there is no need to change bags and empty the drainage each cycle. Furthermore as the number of connections and disconnections is drastically curtailed the chances of peritonitis should be considerably less. However, more time is necessary for staff training and the more sophisticated the equipment the more essential it becomes to avoid a high staff turnover or the investment will be wasted.

Section B

LONG-TERM PERITONEAL DIALYSIS

Introduction

This section is concerned with the use of the Silastic catheter. The problems discussed are those directly relevant to the dialysis procedure or cannula. More general issues such as bone disease are not included. The manual covers problems relevant to CAPD or intermittent manual PD. It does not consider specific events related to machine assisted dialysis, e.g. reversed osmosis or cycler machines, as these are covered in the relevant manufacturer's technical bulletins.

Some of the topics are identical to those encountered with temporary dialysis. In such cases the page will direct the reader to the relevant heading in Section A. As in Section A there is a certain amount of deliberate duplication.

Index for section B

Exit site infection
Tunnel infection
Cannula appears through skin
Cloudy fluid
Peritonitis
Relapsing peritonitis
Antibiotic dosage
Presence of cells in the dialysate
Contamination accidents
Cracked or distorted connector
Split cannula
Re-use of catheter components
Fluid will not run in
Fluid will not run out
Rotation of a faulty catheter
    position
Cannulogram
Fluid balance
Failure to remove excess fluid
Hydrothorax

Oedema of abdominal wall or
    genitalia
Hypotension
Hypertension
Dialysis with a stoma
Peritoneal adhesions and sclerosis
Insertion via laparotomy
Dialysis after laparotomy
Hypokalaemia
Obesity
Lack of subcutaneous fat
Backache
Temporary stopping
Hernia
Baths, showers, swimming
Use of insulin
How many cycles?
Choice of volume
Choice of antiseptic
Heating the fluid

Selection of cannula

A number of different Silastic cannulae are commercially available. They may have one or two cuffs. They may be straight or have a coil. They may be radio-opaque. They can vary in length. Other catheters are available and are said to reduce the chances of omental wrapping (Figure B1).

Detailed comparisons are difficult. However, whatever type is chosen it should have a radio-opaque stripe or be radio-opaque. For small children a special length should be obtained but it is still advisable to have an adult size Dacron cuff to ensure that the catheter stays secure without leakage. As a guide the intra-abdominal portion of the cannula should be the same length as the distance between the umbilicus and the pubis. It is recommended that there should be at least 2 cm of side holes. This means that adult type catheters can be used suitably trimmed in many children. For the very young only one cuff need be used, positioned just above the peritoneal entry point. A subcutaneous tunnel of several centimetres is constructed as usual.

Most units use the standard two cuff straight cannula. Either the straight or the coiled cannula can be inserted via the standard trocar under local anaesthetic. Other catheters usually require a general anaesthetic for placement via laparotomy.

Trolley setting for Silastic catheter insertion

Top shelf	Catheter pack
Bottom shelf	Cannula in its box
	No. 11 scalpel
	No. 24 scalpel
	Silk suture
	Catgut suture
	Povidone-iodine
	Antibiotic spray
	Lignocaine 2%
	Quill
	2 x No. 21 gauge needles
	2 x 20 ml syringes
	Non-stick dressing
	Elastoplast
	Long 15 gauge needle

Separate Trolley   Mask
                         Theatre cap
                         Sterile gown
                         Sterile gloves

Dialysis fluid set up on giving set with drainage bag attached.

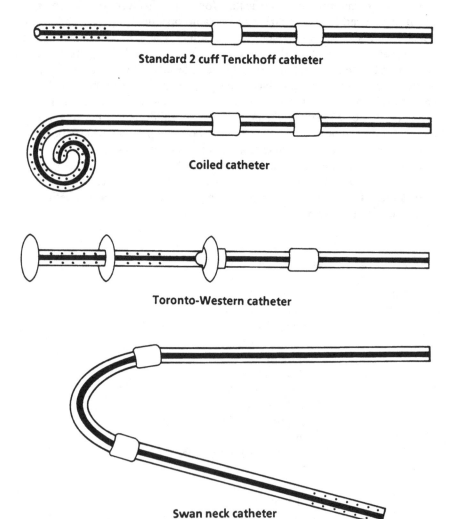

Standard 2 cuff Tenckhoff catheter

Coiled catheter

Toronto-Western catheter

Swan neck catheter

Figure B1 Common types of Silastic catheter. Note radio-opaque stripe along length of each catheter. Not to scale

Contents of Silastic catheter set

4 dressing towels
1 kidney dish
1 gallipot
4 towel clips
1 Tenckhoff type trocar set
1 catheter obturator
1 small self-retaining retractor
2 mosquito straight artery forceps
2 mosquito curved artery forceps
1 toothed dissecting forceps
1 non-toothed dissecting forceps
1 Mayo 5" flat scissors
1 Mayo 5" curved scissors
1 Kilner needle holder
1 pliable uterine sound
Swabs
1 set of dilators
1 tunnelling instrument

Insertion of Silastic catheter   D

This should be done in a clean area preferably in an operating theatre. Both the abdominal skin and the peritoneum must be free of infection.

1.   Explain to patient the procedure and the reasons for catheter insertion. Ensure bladder is empty.
2.   Patient lies with just one or two pillows on operating table. Patient wears a mask.
3.   Patient's abdomen is shaved to just above pubis.
4.   Operator wears cap, mask, sterile gown and sterile gloves. All other personnel wear masks.
5.   Cleanse the abdomen with povidone-iodine. Pay particular attention to the umbilicus and any old puncture sites.
6.   Cover with sterile dressing towels just leaving small area below umbilicus exposed.
7.   Infiltrate linea alba about 3 cm below the umbilicus with local anaesthetic going right to base of the subcutaneous tissue (Figure B2.1). Anaesthetise an area about 5 cm long and 3 cm wide. (This allows for the skin stitches.)

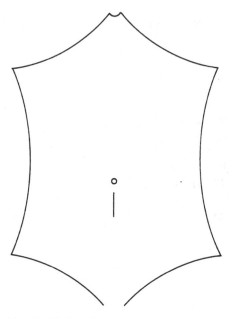

Figure B2.1 Site of incision for Silastic catheter

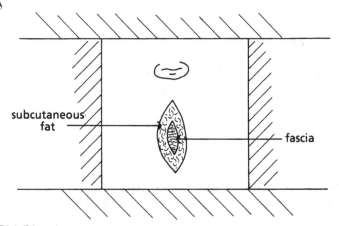

Figure B2.2 Dissection down to linea alba

8. Using No. 24 scalpel incise about 3 to 4 cm of skin over the linea alba starting about 2 cm below the umbilicus.
9. With blunt dissection work down to the linea alba itself securing any bleeding points on the way (Figure B2.2). The self-retaining retractor can be used if necessary but remove it before inserting the cannula as it is otherwise difficult to free.

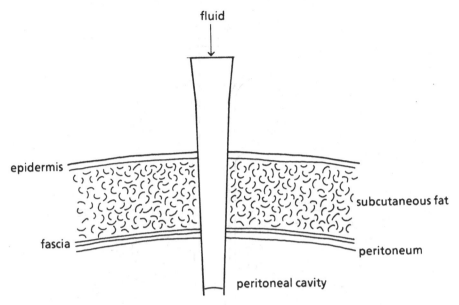

Figure B2.3 Filling abdomen via 15 gauge plastic cannula

10.   Infiltrate small amount of local anaesthetic into linea alba. Insert 15 gauge needle with plastic cannula into peritoneal cavity. Remove needle. Run 1 litre of heparinised dialysate into abdomen (Figure B2.3).

11.   Soak Silastic catheter in PD fluid. Squeeze cuffs in fluid to expel trapped air.

12.   Discard plastic cannula.

13.   Assemble the trocar. Make a small 0.25 cm incision in the linea alba over 15 gauge entry point.

14.   Fit the catheter over the obturator. Check it slides into the trocar.

15.   Insert trocar point into incision in linea alba. Ask the patient to tense the abdomen by bending the head forward. Perforate the peritoneum with the trocar in the vertical position. The patient can then relax (Figure B2.4).

16.   The thin part of the trocar should now be intraperitoneal but the fat part is sitting on the linea alba. Remove the trocar stylet. Fluid will usually be seen inside the trocar lumen. If not, use the catheter obturator to check, gently, that there is no resistance just beyond the trocar tip. If there is, the assembly may still be pre-peritoneal and a new site must be used.

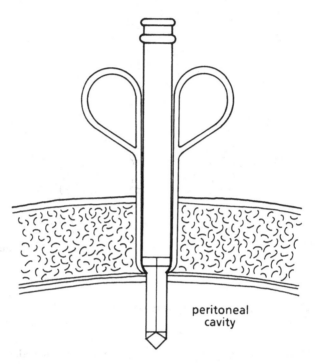

peritoneal
cavity

Figure B2.4 Insertion of assembled trocar

17. The catheter on its obturator is slid through the trocar. Once it has entered the peritoneal cavity the outer end of the assembly is tilted towards the patient's head so that the catheter is pointing down to the pelvis (Figure B2.5).

18. The catheter is slowly advanced, stopping if there is any resistance or pain. If it does not go in satisfactorily it may be withdrawn and reinserted at a different angle.

19. The inner cuff will stick in the assembly at the end of the wide section preventing further insertion. The catheter obturator is then removed. Holding the handles of the narrow part of the trocar firmly, the wide section is slowly removed using a rotating motion to get over the cannula.

20. Holding the cannula in position the two halves of the tip of the trocar are then removed. NB. Their edges are very sharp.

21. Check the catheter patency by gently syringing. Then clamp the catheter to prevent further leakage of dialysate. Ensure the inner cuff is sitting snugly on the linea alba.

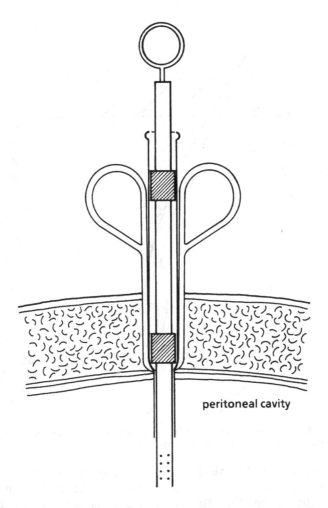

peritoneal cavity

Figure B2.5 Insertion of cannula through trocar. Note how inner Dacron cuff sits in lower end of main trocar body and thus will lie on fascia at end of procedure. The catheter obturator is not allowed to protrude from inner (peritoneal) end of cannula

22. Lay the cannula in a straight line up the abdomen, just missing the umbilicus. Note where the outer cuff lies and mark a point at least 2 cm further towards the head. This will be the skin exit (Figure B2.6).

23. Infiltrate local anaesthetic at this exit point and back down in a straight line in the subcutaneous tissue to the mid-line incision. Infiltrate back up from the incision.

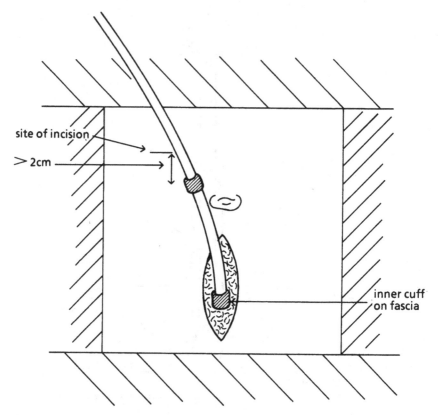

site of incision

> 2cm

inner cuff
on fascia

Figure B2.6 Finding the optimum exit site. Note how the site for the exit is at least 2 cm beyond the outer cuff when this is laid on the abdomen

24. Using a No. 11 scalpel make a small incision about 0.5 cm length over the exit site. Insert a probe through the incision and into the subcutaneous fat. The probe is then passed back to the mid-line incision under the skin coming out near the cephalic end of the wound (Figure B2.7).

25. Make an opening in the subcutaneous fat around the probe wide enough to take the cuff. Sometimes the subcutaneous tissue seems quite fibrous holding up passage of the cuff. It is helpful to widen the tunnel created by the probe but not nearer than 2 cm to the exit site.

26. Secure the catheter end to the probe and pull through the tunnel. The catheter should then be lying in a smooth curve from the inner cuff into the tunnel with no kinks. The subcutaneous portion should be fairly straight.

tunneller

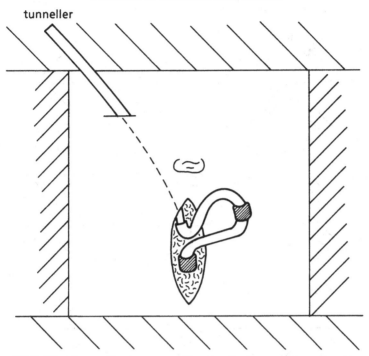

Figure B2.7 Use of tunnelling instrument. The tunneller is passed down from the exit site subcutaneously emerging from the upper end of the insertion wound. The cannula is threaded over the tunneller which is then pulled back

27.   The mid-line incision is closed using catgut for the subcutaneous tissues. A snug fit around the catheter reducing the cavity as much as possible decreases the chance of leakage. Remember that the catheter is not self-sealing so do not puncture. Antibiotic spray can be used if necessary.
28.   Close the skin with silk (Figure B2.8).
29.   If the exit site incision is too big it can be narrowed with one silk stitch but be careful not to pierce the cannula. Insert connector.
30.   Clean the wounds and dry. Apply non-stick dressing (such as Melolin) and then gauze swabs. Cover with elastoplast. This helps to secure cannula.
31.   Connect to dialysis tubing set. Tape junction to prevent disconnection.
32.   Commence dialysis. Subsequently, try to secure the external portion of the catheter so that the inevitable tugging during dialysis does not pull on the cuffs. This will reduce the chance of cuff erosion or leakage.
33.   Stitches may be removed from 7 to 10 days later.

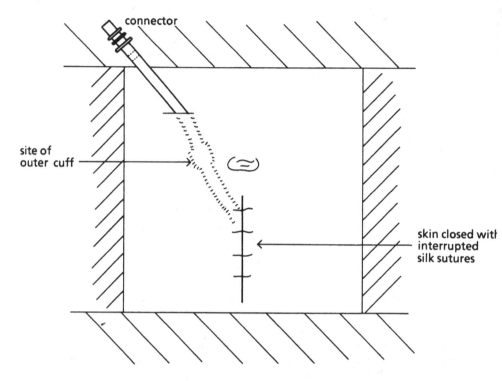

Figure B2.8 Closure of wound. The plastic connector is inserted and dialysis with low volumes can commence immediately

Additional notes   **D**

If necessary a purse string suture can be inserted in the linea alba around the cannula. The cannula can be retained in position by a securing stitch from the linea alba through the Dacron on the inner cuff. Be careful not to puncture the cannula. These measures are more likely to be necessary if the patient is elderly with loose tissues.

A tunnel can be made using a set of dilators. The three smallest are passed up from the mid-line through the skin at the exit site. The three largest are used to dilate the track only as far as the site of the outer cuff, i.e. at least 2 cm from the exit. The third smallest dilator is then passed back down the tunnel. The cannula is slipped over the end of the dilator which is then withdrawn pulling the cannula with it.

Alternatively a commercially available tunnelling instrument can be used. This technique is identical to that described in steps 22 to 24.

Many units use a relatively straight or slightly curved tunnel so that the cannula exits above the umbilicus. It is claimed that a tunnel curving through 180° so that the exit site faces towards the pubis is associated with less chance of exit site infection. This requires the use of a specially curved cannula.

Alternative sites   D

It is possible to insert a Silastic catheter lateral to the linea alba. The best alternative is to place the inner cuff in the rectus sheath. The incision is made just below the umbilicus starting in the mid-line and going laterally for 4-5 cm (Figure B3.1). After dissection down to the rectus sheath a 1 cm incision is made in it in the same direction as the skin cut (Figure B3.2). The fibres of the rectus muscle are separated using a small artery forceps spreading the jaws in the same direction as the incisions (Figure B3.3). The abdomen is then filled with fluid. A catgut suture is placed through each end of the rectus sheath incision and left loose (Figure B3.4). The catheter is inserted in the usual manner. After withdrawing the halves of the trocar, the inner cuff is grasped with forceps and manoeuvred into the sheath between the muscle fibres (Figure B3.5). The catgut sutures are then tied individually closing the sheath over the cuff (Figure B3.6). This produces a very secure and almost always watertight system. The tunnel is constructed in the normal way.

The major disadvantage of this technique is that it is harder to remove the cannula once inserted.

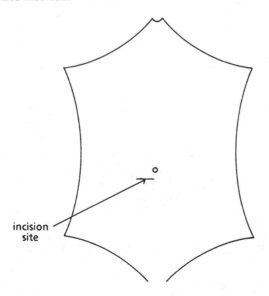

Figure B3.1 Insertion via rectus sheath. An incision 4 cm long is made as indicated

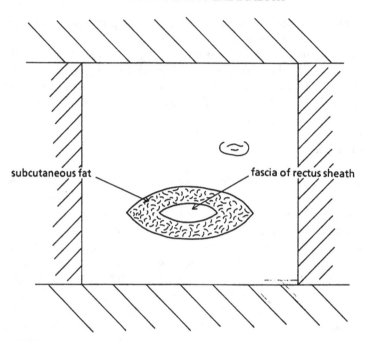

Figure B3.2 Exposure of rectus sheath

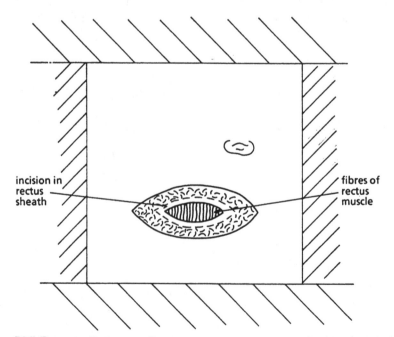

Figure B3.3 Exposure of rectus muscle

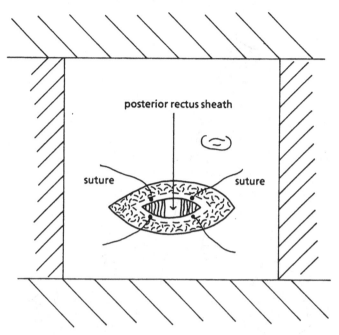

Figure B3.4 Preparation for insertion. Note how the rectus fibres have been separated exposing the posterior rectus sheath. Two sutures have been placed in the anterior sheath ready for closure

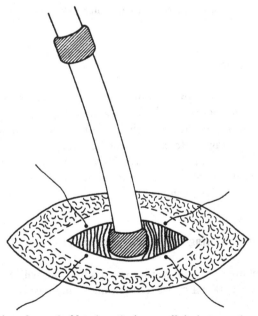

Figure B3.5 Insertion of cannula. Note how the inner cuff sits between the muscle fibres

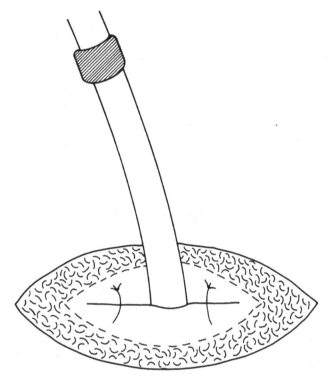

Figure B3.6 Closure of rectus sheath. Note how the sutures close the sheath above the inner cuff

Laparoscopic placement   D

It is possible to insert a cannula using a modified laparoscope, the Needle-scope. The advantages of this technique are that the catheter is guaranteed to be intra-abdominal and in the best pelvic position. The procedure is claimed to have a lower leakage rate and better cannula life than the standard technique though this remains to be confirmed. The equipment is expensive but if it reduces early complications including the need for laparotomy it may prove cost-saving in the long run.

Dialysis procedure following Silastic catheter insertion   D

Start with low volumes. For an average sized adult who will eventually have 2 litre cycles start with 500 ml cycles. Do not allow any dwell. Heparinise each cycle (500 units per litre). Cycles can be continuous or 12 hourly as required by the patient's condition. After 4 days increase volume to 1000 ml each cycle but avoid any dwell. Use 1.36% or 3.86% dextrose as necessary. Similarly add potassium as necessary. 8-10 days after catheter insertion the catheter may safely be capped off for 2-3 days if there have been no problems. Two litre cycles may start, including a CAPD dwell if wished, 12 to 14 days post-insertion. Heparin is not required for most patients after the first week.

Patients should have bed rest for 2 days after insertion and then be allowed to sit out. Straining, coughing and other exertion should be avoided if possible until 10 days. This reduces the chances of a leak occurring.

The wound may be left for 3 days unless there is much pain or bleeding. Subsequently daily dressings are performed. See section on exit site care. Stitches are removed at 10 days.

Alternative procedure following Silastic catheter insertion

Some units do not commence dialysis immediately. Instead, 50 ml of saline containing heparin 1000 units are infused down the catheter every 6 to 12 hours for 5 days when dialysis commences. This technique reduces the chance of a leak but means haemodialysis, usually via a subclavian catheter, has to be used if dialysis is necessary in the interim.

Alternatively after overnight dialysis to check cannula is working satisfactorily disconnect tubing set and cap off. Leave abdomen empty for 7 to 10 days. CAPD can then be commenced without the need for further flushing cycles. This technique reduces the chances of leakage and/or infection.

Exit site care

After cannula insertion the dressing around the exit site should be left for about 3 days unless there is excessive oozing of blood. Following the 3 days the dressing is removed, any clots are sponged away using swabs soaked in povidone-iodine. The area is dried thoroughly and then a piece of gauze is folded under the cannula. Another is placed on top and then taped down. The cannula itself *should be taped to the skin to prevent pulling* on the cuffs before they are secure. This dressing is then repeated every other day including cleansing with povidone-iodine.

Once the patient is home opinions differ on the best procedure. Many units advise daily dressing exactly as described above. Others leave the site uncovered and only perform a dressing including the cleansing with povidone-iodine after a shower or swimming. It has been suggested that cleansing with soap and water alone is sufficient. Whichever technique is used it is essential that the site be left clean and dry.

Prior to all exit site dressings the patient and/or helper should put on a mask and wash hands thoroughly.

Cannula removal   **D**

This should be done in as clean an area as possible preferably in an operating theatre. The patient should wear a mask. The operator must wear a hat, mask, sterile gown, and sterile gloves.

1. Drain out any fluid in the abdomen then clamp cannula.
2. Cleanse old insertion wound, skin exit and area over outer cuff with povidone-iodine.
3. Cover abdomen with sterile towels, leaving insertion wound exposed.
4. Infiltrate with local anaesthetic. Remember to infiltrate alongside where inner cuff is lying.
5. Incise old wound with scalpel. Using blunt dissection locate cannula.
6. The cannula will be found lying in a dense sheath and the cuff will be held by very strong fibrous tissue. Open sheath around cannula.
7. Clamp exposed cannula and retract to bring inner cuff up.
8. Open cannula sheath until cuff edge seen.
9. Trim fibrous tissue off the cuff. This will require blunt dissection and sometimes the use of a scalpel. Be careful not to cut across cannula. Work slowly around cuff until it is free.
10. Withdraw cannula from abdomen and cut off at entry to subcutaneous tunnel. Cut off tip of catheter and send for culture.
11. Sew up the hole in the deep fascia. If there is any worry regarding possible hernia formation consider using a non-absorbable suture but only if there is no infection present.
12. Close subcutanous tissues with catgut and skin with silk.
13. Infiltrate local anaesthetic around outer cuff.
14. Incise longitudinally with scalpel over cuff. If the cuff is close to the skin exit then slit back from exit hole over the cuff.
15. Using blunt dissection and if necessary the scalpel, free the outer cuff.
16. Withdraw inner portion of cannula. If the skin exit has been slit then the remaining portion will come free. Discard, saving connector (see section on re-use).
17. If the outer cuff incision does not meet the skin exit, cut the cannula flush with exit hole and then withdraw entire subcutaneous portion. Discard. Recycle connector on external portion and discard the

catheter itself. This technique minimises the chances of introducing infection from the exterior portion.

18. Close skin of outer cuff incision with silk. Do not try to occlude the exit hole itself.

19. Apply non-stick dressings and cover with gauze swabs and tape.

NB. If either wound is infected *do not* attempt to suture but puff in antibiotic powder and then pack. Infected wounds must be left to heal by granulation. No attempt should be made to insert a further Silastic catheter until such healing has occurred.

Trolley setting for catheter removal

Cut down set
Povidone-iodine
Local anaesthetic
20 ml syringe
21 gauge needle
Scalpel blade
Quill
Universal container
Catgut suture
Silk suture
Antibiotic spray
Non-stick dressing (e.g. Melolin)
Elastoplast or tape

Insertion of a replacement catheter   **D**

The abdomen must be free of infection both in the skin and the peritoneal cavity before a Silastic catheter is replaced. The technique is similar to that used for introducing the original cannula and can be combined with catheter removal if no infection is present. As always the peritoneal cavity should be filled with dialysate prior to insertion using the old cannula if still present. The exit hole should be the opposite side of the abdomen to the original hole. The new catheter can enter the peritoneal cavity via the same hole but check that the hole itself is not too lax. If necessary purse string the linea alba around the new catheter to make a snug fit not occluding the cannula. Hopefully, this will prevent any hernia formation.

Pre-peritoneal placement   **D**

If a cannula is inserted under local anaesthetic it is possible to inadvertently position it in front of the peritoneal cavity. This happens when the trocar has not penetrated the peritoneum. One possible cause is that the fluid has formed a false space under the deep fascia. Running in fluid may well be painful if the tip of the cannula is not inside the peritoneal cavity. Usually the cannula cannot be inserted to any depth and probing with the introducer fails to find a passage down into the pelvis. Outflow is poor or non-existent. If the catheter has actually been inserted in a pre-peritoneal position a lateral X-ray of the abdomen will confirm it does not dip down into the pelvis and a cannulogram will show it is lying in a small space. The treatment is to remove the catheter and either use a different site or replace using a laparotomy. Alternatively laparoscopic placement will guarantee an intra-peritoneal position.

Changing the bag - general advice

The exact technique for changing the bag depends on the CAPD system being used. All manufacturers provide detailed literature relevant to their own products and will arrange in-house training if requested. There is one overriding principle, namely that a no-touch procedure should be used. This means that the parts of the bags and tubing set which physically connect should be regarded as sterile and should not come into contact with hands, table top, swabs etc. It is particularly important that the internal part of the fluid pathway should not be contaminated. If there is a break in the sterile technique then appropriate steps should be taken. See section on contamination accidents.

Procedure for bag change (Baxter spike system)

1. Soak two bag clamps in chlorhexidine (Hibitane) changed every day. Run out fluid.
2. Switch off roller clamp.
3. Wash hands with chlorhexidine scrub (Hibiscrub).
4. Wipe down table top which is to be used for bag change, removing all dirt, dust and stains, with alcohol wipe (Sterets Alcowipe).
5. Open new bag onto table top and check:
    a. date of expiry
    b. volume

     c. concentration of fluid
     d. is tag in place?
     e. is the fluid clear?
     f. is the bag leaking?

6.   Put bag on table with port facing upwards.
7.   Open connector shield packet.
8.   Wash hands again thoroughly and dry in a clean towel. Put mask on.
9.   Place old bag on table top next to the new bag.
10.   Pull new bag blue cover down but not off and put on clamp.
11.   Remove old connector shield.
12.   Put clamp on port of old bag.
13.   Put on a clean pair of gloves and wash with chlorhexidine alcohol (Hibisol).
14.   Hold handle of clamp and pull blue cover off new bag.
15.   Holding handle of clamp pull spike out from old bag and, in one swift movement, being very careful not to touch the end of the spike, put spike into the port of the new bag. While holding the handle of the clamp push spike right into port.
16.   Remove clamp.
17.   Fix connector shield in position without touching the actual junction of bag and line.
18.   Hang bag up and run fluid in.
19.   When fluid has run in clamp line with roller clamp. Take bag off stand and roll bag and line up comfortably with spike inside the bag. Place bag in usual wearing position.
20.   Measure fluid in old bag and record it on your chart.
21.   Replace clamps in chlorhexidine.

If by accident you touch the spike of the line or drop it on the floor, soak it in povidone-iodine for 5 minutes before carrying on with the procedure.

Bag change Baxter system II using 'K' shield *(1st bag of the day only)*

Equipment
     Alcoholic chlorhexidine (Hibisol)
     'K' shield
     Clamps x 2 soaking in chlorhexidine gluconate
     Warm bag

Procedure
1.   Wash hands.

2.   Drain fluid.

3.   Switch off roller clamp.

4.   Clean table top using hard surface disinfectant. Remove all dust.

5.   Assemble equipment on table top
- new bag
- clamps, soaking in pink tincture
- new shield
- Hibisol

6.   Wash hands using 3 applications of chlorhexidine scrub (Hibiscrub). Wash between fingers, around wrists and the backs of the hands!

7.   Dry hands using disposable towel (kitchen roll).

8.   Pick up drip stand with clean disposable towel return to bag change table.

9.   Open new bag. If outer bag intact, check six things:
a. date of expiry
b. volume
c. concentration of fluid
d. is tag in place?
e. is the fluid clear?
f. is the bag leaking?

10.   Open new shield. Ensure that it is moist - do not remove from package.

11.   Open clamp box.

12.   Place clamp on line whilst bag is still on stand.

13.   Lift old bag on to table top.

14.   Clamp outlet port of bag.

15.   Remove shield.

16.   Hibisol hands.

17.   Put new shield onto connection.

18.   Pull down outlet port on new bag and remove tag.

19.   Grasp ribbed part of outlet port of old bag with your left hand and grip ribbed part of your line with right hand. Unscrew.

20.   Holding ribbed part of line in right hand now take hold of ribbed part of outlet port of new bag in left hand and *immediately* screw together.

21.   Remove clamps and break green seal.

22.   Hang bag up and run fluid in.

23.   Take bag off stand, roll up and place in usual wearing position e.g. pocket.

24.   Measure fluid in old bag and record on chart.

25.   Is fluid clear?

26.   Replace clamps in chlorhexidine.

NB. If by accident you touch the connector of the line or drop it, soak in iodine for 5 minutes before carrying on with procedure.

Remaining bags of the day

Fresh 'K' shield not required (i.e. one shield/24 hour)
Omit steps 10, 15 and 17.

Travenol UVXD bag change

1. Run fluid out into old bag.
2. Prepare table - clean with hard surface disinfectant, place new bag, clamps, alcoholic chlorhexidine (Hibisol) and UVXD on table.
3. Test UVXD. Press test switch on top of chamber, a red light should light up and you should hear a short steady signal. WASH HANDS. (IF YOU DO NOT HEAR AND SEE SIGNALS PHONE NUMBER ON TOP OF CHAMBER).
4. Open new bag checking:
    a. date of expiry
    b. volume
    c. concentration of fluid
    d. is tag in place?
    e. is the fluid clear?
    f. is the bag leaking?
    Clamp outlet part of bag with blue clamp.
5. Place new bag to left of UVXD. Open drawer making sure lever is in INSERT position.
6. Close roller clamp on line, place old bag on table, remove green locking collar, clamp outlet port as close to bag as possible.
7. With one hand hold white plastic base of spike and with other hand slide blue shield away from old bag down the line.
8. Place neck of bag and line connection in drawer.
9. Rotate lever clockwise to remove spike.
10. Remove old bag by holding blue clamp. Clean hands with Hibisol.
11. Insert new bag into drawer and remove tip protector by pulling to right and upwards, before pushing neck of bag right down into the groove.
12. Close drawer and blue ON light should glow.
13. When green INSERT SPIKE light glows and you hear broken tone rotate lever to INSERT position while light is still on.
    YOU HAVE 25-30 SECONDS.
14. Open drawer and remove bag.
15. With one hand hold white plastic base; with other hand slide blue shield over connection. Replace green locking collar.
16. Run fluid in.
Lines to be changed by CAPD nurse each 6-8 weeks.

69

CAPD bag change procedure for Baxter 'O' set

1. Wash hands.
2. Clean table.
3. Assemble equipment on table as shown -
   a. 1 new bag
   b. 1 disconnect cap
   c. 2 connection shields
   d. 1 bag gripper in chlorhexidine
   e. 1 organiser
   f. Alcoholic chlorhexidine (Hibisol)
   g. 'O' set and empty bag
4. Add hypochlorite (Milton) to organiser.
5. Wash hands using three applications of Hibiscrub.
6. Open and check shields and new bag -
   Check:
   - date of expiry
   - any leaks?
   - is it clear?
   - blue tag in place
   - strength
   - volume
7. Check all clamps are closed and place empty bag in drainage position.
8. Remove connection shield from 'O' set.
9. Place both ends in organiser ensuring that the long arm of the set is in right hand side.
10. Hibisol hands.
11. Remove blue tag from new bag.
12. Remove line from RIGHT hand side of organiser, connect to new bag and apply connection shield.
13. Remove disconnect cap from extension set.
14. Connect line to LEFT side of organiser to extension set and apply connection shield.
15. Drain out - opening roller clamp on extension set, and clamp on drainage line.
16. When draining is complete, close the clamp on extension set.
17. Hang up new bag and break green seal.
18. Open clamp on inflow line allowing fluid to run for a count of 15 seconds.
19. Close clamp on drainage line and open clamp on extension set and run fluid in. Then close ALL clamps.
20. Open disconnect cap and clamps.

21. Hibisol hands.
22. Remove connection shield from extension set and return it to packet.
23. Disconnect line and put in LEFT side organiser.
24. Apply new disconnect cap to extension set.
25. Place old full bag onto LEFT side of table and clamp outlet part.
26. Remove connection shield, disconnect line and place in RIGHT side of organiser. Leave both ends for ONE minute.
27. Hibisol hands.
28. Take both lines from organiser and reconnect set to form 'O'.
29. Apply connection shield.
30. Store set and bag for next exchange.

NB. Milton to be renewed each morning. Dissolve Milton tablet in 200 ml of water, fill organiser and top up organiser with this solution throughout day.

Bag change using Baxter Freeline (III)

1. Wash hands and expose your line.
2. Clean table top.
3. Collect equipment:-
   disconnect cap - fresh one each day
   'K' shield
   blue clamp
   alcoholic chlorhexidine (Hibisol)
   fresh bag
   freeline
4. Wash hands thoroughly using three applications of Hibiscrub.
5. Open new bag and check:-
   expiry date
   volume
   concentration e.g. 1.36% or 3.8%
   is it clear?
   are there any leaks?
   is the ring in place?
6. Put blue clamp on neck of bag.
7. Open 'K' shield.
   Open freeline - ensuring it remains on sterile paper.
8. Hibisol hands.
9. Remove paper strap from freeline and close both white gates.
10. Remove ring from new bag.

11. Take spike of line and insert into bag. Keep fingers behind finger guard and be careful not to pierce bag.
12. Remove blue tag from freeline and apply 'K' shield.
13. Remove disconnect cap from your line (discard if necessary; if not place in 'K' shield package for protection).
14. Attach 'K' shielded freeline to your line.
15. Hang fresh bag on hook.
16. Put drainage bag on stand.
17. Open both white gates on freeline then remove blue clamp. Allow fluid to run from fresh bag to drainage bag for 15 seconds.
18. Close white gate on inflow line.
19. Open roller clamp and allow drainage from self.
20. When drainage is completed close outflow white gate. Open inflow white gate.
21. When fresh bag is empty close your roller clamp and inflow white gate.
22. Open disconnect cap if required.
23. Hibisol hands.
24. Remove freeline from your line and apply disconnect cap.
25. Check fluid, measure and dispose of freeline, record details.

Changing the tubing

The exact technique for changing the tubing at the cannula end depends on the CAPD system being used. However, it should include a five minute soak of the connection in povidone-iodine. Each manufacturer will advise on the details for their own system and will usually provide staff training.

If intermittent peritoneal dialysis or machine peritoneal dialysis is being used then connection or disconnection should be performed using the same technique as described for temporary cannulae.

Line change involving Baxter CAPD system

Equipment

Line change pack
2 pairs of sterile gloves
2 straight edged clamps used for subclavian cannulae e.g. Vas-cath soaking in chlorhexidine gluconate
French dressing forceps - sterile
Face masks x 2

Povidone-iodine solution
Hard surface disinfectant
Chlorhexidine scrub (Hibiscrub)
Clock with a second hand
An assistant, e.g. nurse or patient

Procedure
1. Drain PD fluid.
2. Clean a surface with disinfectant and assemble:
fresh line
fresh warm bag
shield
alcoholic chlorhexidine (Hibisol)
3. Wash hands thoroughly and attach line to bag. Prime line.
NB. Do not wet the cotton wool in the protective covering at the end of the line.
4. Hang bag on drip stand. Tape protective covering to bag. Ensure there is no risk of contaminating the end of the line.
5. Clean trolley/suitable surface using a hard surface disinfectant.
6. Open sterile line change pack onto the clean surface. Face mask on nurse and patient.
7. Wash hands for *3 minutes* using Hibiscrub.
8. Open pack and dry hands using one of the paper towels contained in pack.
9. Assistant to open both pairs of sterile gloves and pour povidone-iodine solution into pot ensuring the sterile field is not contaminated.
10. Assistant to remove the cannula exit site dressing and clamp the line to the bag.
NB. Examine cannula. Any holes? Examine exit site. Clean and dry?
11. Nurse to put on a pair of sterile gloves and using the paper which contained the gloves with another paper towel from the pack - place these under the cannula and adaptor to create a sterile field.
12. Having disposed of one of the former swabs, now use the fresh swabs to scrub the titanium adaptor itself for *1 minute*.
13. Using one of these swabs, wrap it around the cannula exit site in order to clean it.
14. Saturate two gauze swabs in the povidone-iodine solution. Squeeze the excess from them and holding the titanium adaptor with one swab wash the cannula from adaptor to skin for *1 minute* with the other swab.
15. Dispose of these swabs and soak adaptor in the pot of povidone-iodine solution for *3 minutes*.

73

16. After 3 minutes wrap the adaptor in a fresh swab.
17. Take the Vas-cath clamp from the chlorhexidine solution and place it on the cannula near the patient.
18. Change gloves.
19. Again using the paper from the fresh gloves and another paper towel create a fresh sterile field under the cannula and connection.
20. Take two sterile swabs, one in each hand, taking hold of the adaptor and the line with these, unscrew the connection.
21. Drop the old line away from the sterile field. Take end of the new line and pull it away from the secured plastic covering.
     NB. Ensure the line end itself is not contaminated.
22. Screw new line tightly onto titanium adaptor.
23. Remove clamp from cannula. Open gate on line and allow fluid to drain into patient.
24. Remove used sterile field and gloves.
25. Wash hands. Clean and dress cannula exit site as usual.
26. Tape line securely to abdomen.

Choice of tubing set

The standard CAPD system involves a single piece of tubing to connect the bag to the catheter. This is sometimes called the transfer set. Recent evidence suggests that a Y type tubing may reduce the chances of peritonitis. This involves connecting the cannula to a short stem to which are attached two long pieces of tubing thus forming a Y. Fresh fluid is run in down one line and the effluent drained out into a presterilised empty bag at the end of the other line. Between bag changes the tubing set is disconnected and the cannula is sealed with a disconnect cap.

The basic principle of Y sets is known as flush before fill. This involves firstly running some of the new fluid straight to the drainage bag for 15 seconds. The dialysate in the abdomen is then drained out. Finally the remainder of the new solution is infused into the peritoneal cavity. The idea is that any bacteria introduced during the various connections will be flushed to the outflow bag and not into the abdomen. As originally described an antibacterial agent such as hypochlorite was used to sterilise the cannula connection but recent reports suggest that this is unnecessary. See the section on the Baxter Freeline set for details of usage of such a system.

Injection technique for adding medication to CAPD fluid

1. Wash hands.
2. Clean work top with hard surface disinfectant.
3. Place on work top CAPD bag, alcoholic chlorhexidine (Hibisol), medication vial and 1 syringe, 2 needles and 2 alcohol wipes for each of the medications to be added.
4. Wash hands using three applications of soap (Hibiscrub).
5. Open CAPD bag and check:
   - volume
   - concentration
   - expiry date
   - any leaks?
   - fluid clear?
   - sterile end intact?
6. Assemble needle and syringe.
7. Wipe the top of the medication vial with one alcohol wipe, then draw up required amount.
8. Change needle - never use the same needle to draw up medication and to inject into the CAPD bag; to do so is to run the risk of infection.
9. Clean hands with alcoholic Hibisol.
10. Wipe injection port with alcohol wipe and inject medication through self sealing rubber cap. Do not let the needle touch your hand, the outside of CAPD bag or the work top.
11. After injection invert CAPD bag and squeeze port to ensure thorough mixing and no leakage.

Sampling

Whenever there is any chance of infection a sample of the outflow must be obtained. It is important to remember that neither the cannula, the tubing nor the bags are self-sealing. The sample *must only be taken* from a rubber insert or entry port. If a manual intermittent system is being used the sample should be taken as described in the appropriate section of the temporary cannula part of this handbook. The hands should be washed and then non-sterile gloves put on. The gloved hands should then be washed with alcoholic chlorhexidine (Hibisol) prior to taking sample. If CAPD is being used then after outflow is complete a sample should be taken via the rubber injection port used for any additives on the bag itself. The rubber must be cleansed with povidone-iodine and without touching the hands a 21 gauge needle on a syringe should be inserted. Fluid may then be aspirated to send to the laboratory. The exact volume necessary depends on individual laboratory requirements.

The tubing set for CCPD cycle machines usually includes a sampling port on the patient connection line.

If a Drake-Willock reversed osmosis machine is in use then the patient line contains a rubber port for aspirating fluid in an identical manner. Aspiration should be performed during outflow, not after it is complete.

See section on when to sample and sampling in temporary cannula part of this manual.

Use of heparin

Heparin should be added to the dialysate at a dosage of 500 units per litre for a week after cannula insertion to prevent it being blocked by clot or fibrin. Subsequently, most patients will not require this drug. If peritonitis should occur exudation may be sufficiently severe that fibrin appears on drainage. Heparin should then be added until the infection has macroscopically cleared. Similarly it is wise to use the drug for a few days after any abdominal operation. Occasionally, patients seem to get a problem with fibrin appearing in the absence of infection. Such patients will require heparin routinely to prevent catheter occlusion. In this situation use of the drug solely in the overnight bag may prove sufficient to solve the problem.

Fibrin in fluid

Strands of fibrin may be seen in the outflow in the first few days after insertion. The use of heparin should prevent cannula occlusion. Subsequently the presence of fibrin may indicate infection and it is essential to culture the fluid even if it otherwise appears clear. Occasional patients may have visible fibrin in their effluent in the absence of infection. Heparin should be used if the system is running slowly. Sometimes just adding the drug to the overnight bag is sufficient to deal with the problem.

Flushing cannula

The technique is similar to that described for a temporary cannula. The catheter should be occluded with an A-V shunt clip or subclavian catheter clamp prior to disconnection from the tubing.

Use of urokinase

Urokinase can be used to try and unblock a cannula which appears to be clogged by fibrin. The technique is the same as that described for a temporary cannula.

Pain in abdomen   **D**

Some pain may occur in the wound for a few days after insertion. This may be relieved by simple analgesics. Subsequently, dialysis with a Silastic catheter should be painless. Should pain in the abdomen occur the most likely cause is infection. The fluid should be inspected. If it is cloudy there is almost certainly infection present. However, if the fluid is clear, though it must be checked bacteriologically, another cause should be sought for the pain. If infection is the cause of the pain then it will disappear when the fluid clears. Occasionally patients seem to have a sore abdomen persisting for a few days after the fluid is macroscopically clear.

It is important not to forget that a fixed or strangulated hernia may be a cause of persistent abdominal pain.

Some patients may feel discomfort or even pain in the abdomen, lower ribs or shoulders, when the fluid is run out. This 'empty sensation' usually occurs in the first few weeks of treatment and tends to disappear with time. If infection is excluded the patient can be reassured and if necessary given a mild analgesic.

Air may also cause pain the first 1-2 weeks after catheter insertion (see section on pain in abdomen with temporary cannula).

Cannulae which allow the abdomen to be filled by 'spraying' may cause less discomfort on running in than a standard one where there is more of a 'jet'.

Bloodstained fluid   **D**

Following insertion of a Silastic catheter the fluid may be bloodstained. This usually clears within a few days. It is wise to add heparin to the dialysate at a concentration of 500 units per litre for the first week. Subsequently, blood in the fluid is uncommon. Occasional patients may have a few bloodstained cycles after being on dialysis for some time, perhaps due to lysis of a clot. Rarely the bleeding may appear to relate to the menstrual cycle. Unless blood loss is significant or infection is present such occurrences are of no serious significance. The fluid should be cultured and heparin added to prevent clotting in the cannula. Persistent and/or severe blood loss indicates the need for a laparotomy to find and secure the bleeding point.

Yellow or orange fluid   D

The longer the dialysate is left in the abdomen the more yellow it will appear on drainage. This is in part due to a slowly increasing protein content and is of no importance.

If the patient becomes jaundiced some of the excess bilirubin will appear in the fluid, colouring it a deep yellow.

Finally taking the drug rifampicin may cause the fluid to appear yellow or orange. This does not matter in itself.

Leakage of fluid   D

It is important to determine the exact site of the leakage. If the fluid is coming from the connecting tubing or bag this must be replaced. If there appears to be a hole or crack in the plastic connector or cannula itself these must be dealt with by replacing or trimming as appropriate. See sections on cracked connector or split cannula.

Sometimes fluid leaks from the abdomen either at the cannula skin outlet or from the mid-line insertion site. Such leakage is usually an early problem after catheter placement. It is made more likely if the patient is mobilised too soon or too large a volume is used early on. Treatment consists of reducing cycle volumes by half and avoiding any dwell times. Sometimes it may be necessary to stop for 12 to 48 hours. When restarting dialysis keep to low volumes for a while, e.g. 500 ml cycles for an average sized adult. If the problem persists then the cannula will need re-exploring. When the old incision is opened the inner cuff will be found to be sitting in a small cavity with a smooth wall. This lining should be trimmed off to provide a granulating surface for the cuff. The same cannula can be used as long as there is no infection. Sometimes it is worth putting a purse string suture in the linea alba around the catheter but avoiding pulling too tightly and thus causing significant occlusion of the cannula lumen.

The chances of leakage are much less if peritoneal dialysis is avoided for 1 week after catheter insertion and/or the inner cuff is placed in the rectus sheath.

Fluid leaks through the vagina   D

A few patients having CAPD have been reported who apparently leaked the dialysate through the vagina. This either occurred via open fallopian tubes or because of a direct fistula from the peritoneal cavity into the vagina. The patients tended to present with peritonitis but also had a watery vaginal discharge with a high glucose content.

Surgical repair of the leak may be feasible but a transfer to haemodialysis should also be considered.

Crusting around cannula

A small amount of crusting may occur at the exit site. If it is not accompanied by redness or pus formation then it is probably not serious. The crusts should be treated daily by soaking in povidone-iodine and gently removed with gauze swabs. A dry dressing should then be placed around the cannula.

If crusting is excessive and/or there is obvious redness then suspect an infection and treat appropriately. See section on entry site infections.

Cuff erosion   D

Sometimes the outer cuff slowly erodes out of the skin. A number of factors may contribute to this problem including exit site infection and placing the cuff too close to the skin surface. Prevention involves ensuring the exterior edge of the cuff is lying at least 2 cm from the skin surface at the exit during insertion. The external portion of the cannula must be secured to prevent the dialysis tubing pulling on the cuff during the first few weeks of dialysis. The actual exit hole in the skin should not be too wide but just snug around the catheter.

If the cuff does start to erode out, provided there is no infection present no urgent measures are necessary. Local cleansing with povidone-iodine and a dry dressing will suffice. However, should most of the cuff appear, a careful watch is necessary to detect any sign of tunnel infection which may require treatment by catheter removal. If the cuff becomes completely free and there is no sign of infection then the cannula can be left in situ if it is otherwise working well.

If cuff erosion is accompanied by exit site infection then early treatment is necessary. See section on exit site infection.

Exit site infection (Figure B4)   **D**

The signs of infection at the exit site are redness, crusting and visible pus.
Sometimes there will be pain and tenderness. A small halo of mild redness on
its own around the cannula up to 0.5 cm is quite common and is not serious.
Slight crusting may also occur with normal cannulae. Anything further
represents infection. Most patients will not be systemically ill. A swab should
be taken for culture. The commonest causative organism is *Staphylococcus
aureus*. Local measures can be tried. These consist of daily or more frequent
cleansing of the site with povidone-iodine, gentle removal of soft or loose
crusts, followed by a dressing. Sometimes an oral antibiotic will be of benefit.

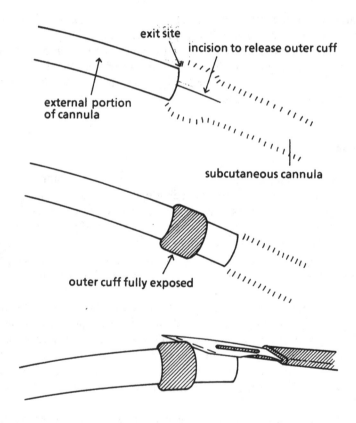

Figure B4 Procedures used to deal with exit site infections. Shave off the outer cuff with a
scalpel. Keep the flat of the blade parallel to the cannula surface

If the outer cuff is visible or close to the surface, it is likely that the infection will not be eradicated but will flare up again. It is then best to exteriorise the cuff by slitting the tunnel to just beyond the cuff under local anaesthetic. The cuff is then placed on top of a small piece of non-stick dressing. The wound usually heals in 2 to 3 weeks. Often the infection will then disappear but if not the only long-term solution may be catheter removal and replacement at a new outlet site under antibiotic cover. Occasionally parenteral vancomycin 1 g i.v. for four doses at weekly intervals may prove effective on its own but care is necessary to avoid reactions due to too rapid infusion. It is claimed that if there is a chronic exit site problem then the removal of the cuff from the catheter by shaving with a scalpel may allow the infection to settle. Great care is necessary to prevent the cannula itself from being perforated.

If the outer cuff totally erodes so that it is no longer attached to the skin the infection may clear up. Should the infection clinically disappear a close watch should be kept but there is no urgent need for catheter replacement.

It has recently been suggested that relapsing exit site infection may respond to a combination of oral flucloxacillin and rifampicin but this has not been confirmed for a large number of affected patients.

Tunnel infection   D

Occasionally infection may occur in the subcutaneous tunnel. This is particularly likely to occur if the outer cuff has come out of the skin. The signs are tenderness and redness over the cannula track and sometimes pus appearing at the exit site. There is a serious risk of peritonitis if this infection is not treated urgently. If the site of infection is not too close to the inner cuff (at least 3 cm away) then deroofing can be tried. Under local anaesthetic the tunnel is slit back from the exit site to just beyond the infected area. The cannula is lifted out and any obvious debris removed. After cleansing the wound it is covered with a non-stick dressing and the cannula laid on top before the gauze swabs are applied. If the infection fails to resolve or is closer to the inner cuff then the cannula must be removed and if the area around the inner cuff is involved it should be packed and not sutured together. Appropriate systemic or oral antibiotics are required. Vancomycin is of value for Gram-positive infections. Dialysis can be continued via a temporary peritoneal catheter inserted the opposite side of the abdomen or by using haemodialysis. When the abdomen is healed and infection-free a new Silastic catheter can be inserted. Haemodialysis is best performed using a subclavian a catheter as this avoids the risk of destroying possible future sites for permanent vascular access.

81

Cannula appears through skin   D

Very rarely a portion of the cannula appears through the abdominal skin. This is most likely to occur through the mid-line incision if the catheter does not lie in a smooth curve but is kinked. The inherent torsion may then force it up before wound healing occurs. An alternative cause is an untreated tunnel infection which bursts through the skin exposing the cannula.

Whatever the cause urgent catheter removal is required. When the abdomen has healed and is free of infection a new cannula can be inserted.

Cloudy fluid   D

The usual cause of cloudy fluid is excess white cells due to infection. Occasionally no organisms are grown. So-called aseptic peritonitis may occur but a discussion with the laboratory is essential to ensure that an energetic search for a pathogen is made.

If nothing is grown but the fluid stays cloudy it is important to exclude other intra-abdominal pathology, particularly inflammatory. Both pseudo-membranous enterocolitis and a localised abscess may cause this clinical picture. Consideration should be given to a laparotomy and/or catheter removal. If the catheter is removed the inner tip must be cultured.

Patients who have recently started on CAPD may have cloudy fluid due to the presence of eosinophils. A differential white count on the deposit will establish this diagnosis. The dialysate should still be cultured but if there is no growth no action is necessary as this condition of eosinophilic peritonitis is usually self-limiting. It is thought to represent an allergic reaction to some constituent(s) of the system.

Peritonitis   D

The single most frequent and most important complication of any form of peritoneal dialysis, but especially CAPD, is peritonitis. Often the first sign is the appearance of cloudy fluid on outflow. Subsequently the patient will have generalised abdominal pain and a temperature. On examination the abdomen will be tender and if untreated guarding and rigidity may occur. Bacteraemia can then ensue as a late complication.

Immediately there is any suspicion of peritonitis a sample of the outflow should be taken (see section on sampling) and sent to the laboratory. A Gram stain should be performed on the spun deposit to guide management. Irrespective of this result cultures should be set up.

Pending sensitivity results the patient should be started on antibiotics based on the likely organisms. If the patient is clearly seriously ill then parenteral antibiotics will be required. However, most patients can be successfully managed just by adding the drugs to the dialysis fluid. Should there be a lot of abdominal discomfort and/or obvious fibrin plugs in the outflow then a few 1-hourly cycles containing heparin should be performed. This will 'flush' out some of the exudate and improve patient comfort. Subsequently the patient can continue on CAPD.

Should a Gram-positive organism be found vancomycin should be given. If a Gram-negative organism is present then an aminoglycoside, e.g. gentamicin, is tried. If both Gram-positive and Gram-negative organisms are seen, or neither, then both antibiotics are given until the culture report is available. Some units recommend a loading dose of antibiotic as well as a maintenance dose to try and ensure adequate tissue levels early on. Recommended doses are given in the section on antibiotics.

Though the use of vancomycin and an aminoglycoside together in the initial treatment of CAPD peritonitis has proved effective for a number of years, there has been some concern about the potential ototoxicity of this combination of drugs. Vancomycin remains the drug of choice for Gram-positive organisms though teicoplanin may prove an acceptable non-ototoxic alternative. Instead of an aminoglycoside a broad spectrum cephalosporin can be used. A further alternative would be vancomycin and aztreonam which has been reported to be effective. Finally one of the newer quinolones such as ciprofloxacin may prove useful but more experience is required before they can be recommended.

To date the standard regime for treating peritonitis has involved antibiotics being administered in each bag while CAPD continues. However several studies have shown that less frequent treatment is possible. For instance, vancomycin is as effective when given intravenously or intraperitoneally as a bolus which is repeated once after 7 days. Such regimes may prove cheaper and involve considerably less work for both patients and staff. At present an i.p. bolus is preferred (see section on antibiotic dosage).

If the patient is not particularly ill then after sampling and receiving the first dose of antibiotic he or she can return home. Many patients can be taught to add antibiotics to the bags themselves but if they or a helper are not proficient a nurse will need to call daily. Most of the recommended antibiotics are stable for up to 24 hours in PD fluid. Thus a nurse (district nurse in the UK) can prepare all four bags with the necessary drugs at one visit.

Once the right antibiotic is given the fluid usually starts clearing within 48 hours. Antibiotics should be given for several days after cultures become negative. How many days is uncertain, but one full week seems effective, i.e. a 10 day course in all.

Should the infection not be controlled within a week then the cannula is contributing to persistence and must be removed. A temporary cannula can be inserted but if the fluid is not sterile in a few days despite continuing lavage with the appropriate antibiotic, then the patient must be transferred to haemodialysis, all peritoneal cannulae removed and systemic antibiotics given. A new Silastic catheter should not be inserted for at least 2 weeks. A few centres have reported replacing Silastic cannulae at the same time as removing the old one with successful eradication of infection by continuing antibiotics, but this method of dealing with resistant peritonitis has yet to find general favour.

If the infection is fungal or due to a yeast, it is possible to sterilise the abdomen with a drug such as amphotericin in the fluid but as this is fungistatic and not cidal it may take up to 4 weeks before cultures are negative and the fluid clear. By then there may be severe adhesions. It is wiser in the presence of a fungal infection to remove the cannula immediately and use haemodialysis for a month before trying a further Silastic catheter. Usually no systemic anti-fungal agent is necessary.

Relapsing peritonitis   D

A relapse is usually defined as the recurrence of peritonitis due to the same organism within 4 weeks of completion of an antibiotic course. If the organism is Gram-positive a combination of i.p. vancomycin and oral rifampicin is recommended for a further 4 weeks. Any additional relapse means the catheter should be removed, and the patient transferred to haemodialysis for 3 weeks. An appropriate antibiotic is given, usually orally. A new cannula can then be inserted.

If relapsing Gram-negative peritonitis occurs then the catheter should be removed. The patient should be treated with appropriate antibiotics i.v. and given haemodialysis for at least 3 weeks before a new PD cannula is inserted. Mixed infections and/or anaerobes strongly suggest a bowel perforation has occurred and an urgent laparotomy is necessary.

Antibiotic dosage for CAPD   D

The table below lists recommended dosages for adding to the dialysate. If necessary a loading dose may be given as indicated. The dosage assumes the patient is maintained on CAPD.

Name	Loading Dose (mg per litre)	Maintenance Dose (mg per litre)
Penicillin	1,000,000 units	50,000 units
Cloxacillin	1000	250
Ampicillin	1000	125
Azlocillin	2000	500
Mezlocillin	2000	500
Piperacillin	4 g i.v. 12 hourly	
Cefuroxime	500	250
Cefotaxime	500	250
Cefoxitin	500	100
Ceftazidine	500	125
Gentamicin	1.7 mg/kg body weight/bag	4-8
Tobramycin	1.7 mg/kg body weight/bag	4-8
Amikacin	100	20
Netilmicin	2.0 mg/kg body weight/bag	5-10
Vancomycin	1000 (intravenously or into bag)	25
alternative	2 doses of 30 mg/kg in bag	
regime	at 7 day intervals	
Amphotericin	Same as maintenance	5
Fusidic acid (see note)	Not known	50
Aztreonam	500	250
Rifampicin	600 mg orally per day	

Note

Penicillins should not be mixed with aminoglycosides in the same bag as they may be inactivated. Cephalosporins and aminoglycosides must not be mixed in the same syringe but can be combined in the same dialysate bag. Clindamycin as marketed in the UK is not recommended for use in dialysate as it requires hydrolysis to become the active drug and therefore will need to be absorbed before it is effective. It is important to check serum levels if patients have aminoglycosides (see antibiotic section for the temporary cannula). Monitoring blood levels is not normally necessary if vancomycin or amphotericin is used i.p.

The dosages for mezlocillin and azlocillin are tentative pending further clinical experience.

It is unwise to use fusidic acid on its own as resistance may develop rapidly.

Though i.v. vancomycin is effective there is a risk of reactions if care is not taken. Thus for routine use the author recommends i.p., either continuous or as a bolus repeated after 7 days.

Additional details on the management of infections during CAPD including antibiotic dosage are given in the literature cited in the further reading list.

Presence of cells in the dialysate   D

The outflow from peritoneal dialysis will contain a few cells but these are not significant. If infection occurs there is a massive outpouring of polymorphs. In fact, if there is no increase in polymorphs any positive culture may well be a false one. (See section on false positive cultures with a temporary cannula.) Usually when infection is significant the number of polymorphs present is sufficient to make the fluid cloudy to the naked eye.

Sometimes during the first few weeks of dialysis eosinophils may be found in substantial numbers. This may represent an allergic reaction to some constituent of the dialysis system. Usually this phenomenon is self-limiting despite continuing dialysis.

If intermittent peritoneal dialysis is used so that there are breaks of 48 hours or more between dialyses then cells may accumulate in the residual fluid. Should this be drained out prior to inflow of new fluid, it may appear cloudy though no infection is present. Microscopically many of the cells will be found to be macrophages but again this is of no serious significance.

Contamination accidents   D

Sometimes there may be a break in the sterile technique. For instance the end of the tubing may be dropped on the floor during a bag change or may miss the entry port and hit the fingers, clamp etc. A leak from the bag, tubing or cannula should be regarded as potential contamination. Any such event should be reported immediately, particularly if it occurs at home. Whatever has happened the dialysis should cease immediately and the patient made to bear down ensuring fluid is flowing out and not in. The system should be clamped at once between the site of contamination and the cannula exit site. If not already in hospital, the patient should report as soon as possible.

At the hospital the relevant contaminated part should be replaced in the standard aseptic manner. If there has been gross contamination the patient should have prophylactic antibiotics in the fluid for 72 hours. Vancomycin and gentamicin in the usual maintenance doses will suffice. Should there be only a slight slip such as just touching the spike on the clamp the relevant part can be cleansed with povidone-iodine for 5 minutes and then dialysis continue. The patient should be advised to report any abdominal pain or cloudiness of the fluid particularly in the next 48 hours. Following a known contamination incident clinical peritonitis does not appear for 24 to 48 hours. After any contamination a review of staff and/or patient techniques must be performed to reduce the chances of a similar event.

The same general rules apply in the event of contamination during intermittent peritoneal dialysis as with CAPD.

It should be noted that though the author recommends prophylactic antibiotics for any significant contamination accident there is as yet no controlled trial proving their efficacy. Furthermore whether oral or intraperitoneal treatment is necessary is also unknown.

Cracked or distorted connector

Occasionally the plastic connector may be cracked. One possible cause is the inadvertent use of a strong clamp. If the connector becomes cracked or distorted it must be changed using an aseptic technique.

1. The cannula should be clamped with a shunt clip and the roller on the tubing closed.
2. The connection to the tubing is then soaked with a swab of povidone-iodine for 5 minutes.
3. The dialysis tubing is disconnected and the end kept covered with a swab soaked in povidone-iodine.
4. The old connector is removed. A new one is then inserted. Insertion is helped if the cannula side of the connector is wetted with povidone-iodine prior to placing in the catheter.
5. The tubing is reconnected. Clamps are removed and dialysis recommences.

Titanium connectors rarely, if ever, get damaged. If they do they should be changed in an identical manner.

Split cannula

Sometimes the Silastic catheter itself may crack or split. There is then a grave risk of peritonitis. It is important to carefully examine the catheter at each clinic visit and also if any infection occurs to exclude small holes. They are particularly likely to occur over or just beyond the connector. The patient usually notices the problem as any dressing or the skin itself becomes wet.

Should any hole or split be found then dialysis must be stopped. Any fluid in the abdomen should be run out and the catheter clamped with an AV shunt clip between the hole and the skin. The patient should then report to hospital immediately if at home. The catheter must be trimmed as follows:

1.   Operator to wear mask and sterile gloves after scrubbing.
2.   Wrap swab soaked in povidone-iodine around area with the hole. Leave for 5 minutes.
3.   Cut cannula with a scalpel just on the skin exit side of the hole.
4.   Discard removed part of cannula. Insert new connector and recommence dialysis.
5.   Take sample for culture.
6.   If the old connector is satisfactory, recycle as described (see section on re-use).
7.   Give prophylactic antibiotics pending culture report. These can be stopped after 3 days if culture was negative and no overt peritonitis ensues.

This procedure can be performed by a trained nurse.

If the extra-abdominal portion of the catheter becomes excessively short it is possible to re-extend the length using a commercially available kit.

Re-use of catheter components

The catheter itself cannot be re-used but several parts of the connecting system can be re-cycled. The rubber cap can be used many times as long as it still fits securely. For intermittent dialysis it can either be sterilized by immersion in a container of povidone-iodine or autoclaved. The titanium connectors for CAPD are virtually indestructible. If they are not obviously warped, after thorough cleansing they may be autoclaved.

The plastic connector normally supplied with the catheter is used for intermittent forms of dialysis. Sometimes it may crack and require replacement. However, it is possible to re-cycle these connectors from cannulae which have to be removed. The connector should be carefully inspected to ensure there is no crack or distortion. It then requires thorough cleansing and can then be autoclaved.

The rubber caps, titanium and plastic connectors can be purchased separately. Separate connecting systems for intermittent dialysis can be obtained commercially.

Fluid will not run in

A 2 litre bag of fluid normally takes about 15 minutes to run into the abdomen. More than 30 minutes is abnormal. Should there be a problem with inflow check the roller clamp is not closed. Make sure the tubing is not kinked, particularly under clothing. Ensure the cannula is not kinked. Sometimes an air lock prevents inflow. Squeezing the bag will usually overcome this cause of fluid not running in. Bags containing a frangible seal should be checked to see if this has been broken properly. If these simple measures fail the cannula should be aseptically flushed. If the cannula then becomes patent, and particularly if bits of fibrin are obtained, heparin should be added to the dialysate for a few days at a concentration of 500 units per litre. Failure to obtain a good inflow despite flushing is an indication for a plain X-ray to show the catheter position. If it is in the pelvis an attempt to clear it with urokinase should be made. Success once again means the dialysate requires added heparin for a few days. If the catheter is in the wrong position or cannot be cleared it will require replacement or rotation. See next section.

Fluid will not run out

Normally, 2 litres run out in about 30 minutes. More than 60 minutes is abnormal. Should there be a problem with outflow ensure the roller clamp is undone and the tubing is free with no kinks in the catheter. Get the patient to strain for a few seconds to overcome any air lock. Make sure the bag is well below the level of the abdomen to maximise the syphon effect. Sometimes, changing body position may help matters. Very occasionally running a further 1 litre into the abdomen may be followed by a good outflow. Check if the patient is constipated and treat with a gentle enema if necessary. This will sometimes get outflow going. If these measures fail, the cannula should be flushed aseptically. Should this re-establish outflow then add heparin for a few cycles to the dialysate. If outflow is still poor then take a plain X-ray of the abdomen to check on the catheter position (Figures B5 and B6). Assuming it is in the pelvis, try freeing with urokinase. If this fails the catheter may well be trapped by omentum producing a one-way valve effect. A cannulogram may be of value to help diagnose this problem. A faulty position and/or omental wrapping requires catheter replacement or rotation. When the omentum is causing the problem it is often better to remove it at laparotomy and ensure the catheter is placed in the pelvis under direct vision. Alternatively the omentum can be stitched up out of the way. This has the advantage of securing the tissue in case it is required for help in repairing a urinary leak after a transplant.

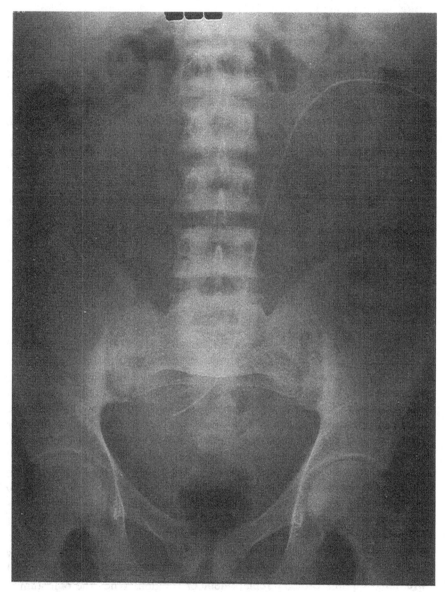

Figure B5 Plain X-ray of abdomen. The radio-opaque stripe on the cannula can be clearly seen and the tip is lying in the pelvis. In this position dialysis should function satisfactorily

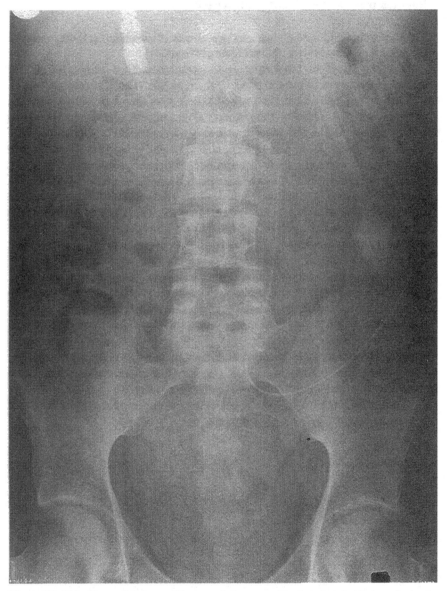

Figure B6 Plain X-ray of abdomen. The cannula has curved back so that the tip is at the level of the iliac crest. This was caused by omental wrapping and required surgery for correction

Rotation treatment of a faulty catheter position   **D**

The following technique is suggested as a means of avoiding catheter renewal when malposition is the problem (Figures B7 and B8).

The procedure involves rotating the catheter with a semi-rigid rod. A suitable instrument is the introducer for a cannula. The end must be round and the whole instrument is sterilised. The rod is then bent into a curve to accommodate the curve of the catheter going into the abdomen. Using an aseptic technique the introducer is slowly and gently slid down the lumen of the catheter under X-ray screening control. If it will not go into the abdomen it is withdrawn and the curve refashioned. Different positions are tried but excessive force must not be used. Once the rod is well inside the abdomen the handle is grasped and pushed gently down the cannula. Sometimes the catheter will be seen to slip back down into the pelvis as the introducer is advanced. If not then rotate the introducer slowly. Several turns may be necessary (maximum six in one direction). The procedure should be stopped if there is any pain, or screening shows bowel is moving with the catheter. If the catheter moves freely it is moved back to a more satisfactory position and then inflow and outflow are re-checked. Failure to rotate and/or correct the original problem with the dialysis means the catheter will require to be repositioned surgically. If the problem recurs then a laparotomy and possible omentectomy will be necessary.

If the cannula curves into the abdomen sharply, forming almost a right angle, then the introducer will be unable to pass down the tunnel and negotiate the bend. Laparotomy will then be necessary.

This procedure should only be performed by a doctor experienced in the routine insertion of Silastic PD catheters.

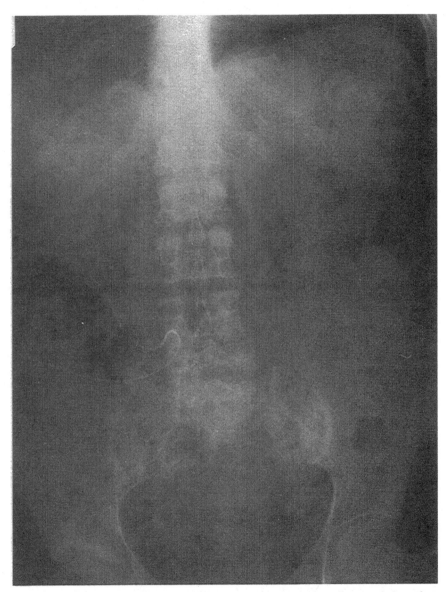

Figure B7 Plain X-ray of abdomen. The cannula has swung laterally several days after placement in the pelvis. Rotation under screening satisfactorily repositioned this catheter

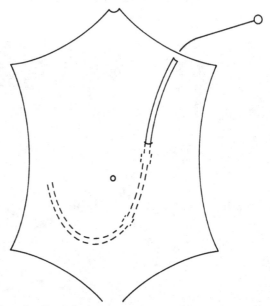

Figure B8.1 Rotation of catheter in faulty position. Tenckhoff cannula obturator with a smooth curve at inner end ready to slide down cannula

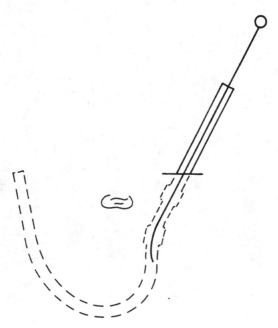

Figure B8.2 Advancement of obturator. Under X-ray screening the obturator is now seen to have just entered the peritoneal cavity

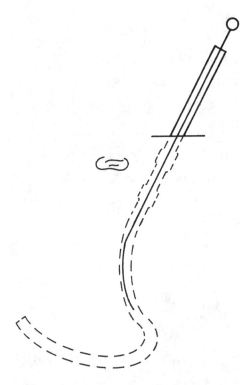

Figure B8.3 Repositioning of catheter in pelvis. As obturator is slowly advanced the catheter will often slip back down into the pelvis

Cannulogram   **D**

It is sometimes necessary to determine why a cannula is not functioning properly. The use of cannulae with a radio-opaque stripe is a considerable help. A plain X-ray of the abdomen will show if the catheter is in the pelvis or has become misplaced. If it is obviously pointing high up in the abdomen then no further investigation is necessary as the only definite solution is surgical repositioning though rotation may be feasible (see section on fluid will not run out and rotation treatment). If it is in the right position but not functioning properly then a cannulogram may be of value. Radio-opaque dye is infused from a syringe down the cannula using aseptic techniques. It is then possible to see if the dye flows freely from the holes into the peritoneal cavity or whether the catheter appears to be encased, implying fibrin or omental trapping (Figure B9). If the catheter appears trapped or encased it will

95

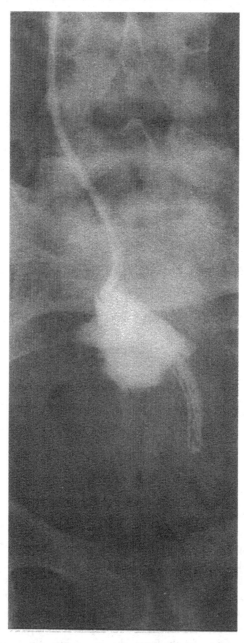

Figure B9 Cannulogram. The radio-opaque dye is filling a small cavity. Normally it should outline loops of bowel. In this example the cannula had been placed inadvertently in a pre-peritoneal position

probably have to be surgically freed. Where the omentum seems to be causing the trouble then it is often better for a laparotomy to be performed, the omentum removed or stitched out of the way and the same or a new cannula placed under direct vision into the pelvis. In this way the problem will not recur.

Fluid balance   D

As with any patient suffering from renal failure, the fluid balance of patients having long-term peritoneal dialysis is best assessed by daily weighing. If CAPD is used the weight should not change much over a week. However, because of the dextrose being absorbed from a CAPD system some patients may slowly gain weight over the months due to fat rather than fluid. Patients having intermittent peritoneal dialysis will have weight gains between treatments similar to those experienced by haemodialysis patients. Gains in excess of 2 kg for an average size adult between any two consecutive treatments mean excessive fluid intake.

All patients will require some fluid restriction, even those receiving CAPD. To try and prevent excessive dextrose absorption it is best if patients have a maximum of one 3.86% dextrose bag per 24 hours. The fluid intake should be restricted appropriately.

Failure to remove excess fluid   D

It is common experience that ultrafiltration decreases if there is peritonitis. Sometimes the patient will notice that he/she removes less fluid for up to 24 hours before presenting with an obvious infection. While peritonitis is present use of bags with more dextrose may not be successful in removing fluid. Once the infection is controlled ultrafiltration returns to normal.

If infection is not the cause of the difficulty then a number of measures can be tried. Initially increasing to two 3.86% bags a day may be helpful but usually the patient has tried this before seeking help. Next an extra 3.86% bag should be used first thing in the morning with a short dwell time of 30-60 minutes. This is often effective as a considerable part of the excess fluid removed by ultrafiltration is present in the abdomen within half an hour of inflow. In addition if the patient is passing any urine then large doses of Frusemide may help fluid balance. Should the problem be more severe then a switch to intermittent dialysis using alternative 1.36% and 3.86% cycles should be tried. Finally if the patient has pulmonary oedema and peritoneal dialysis does not rapidly remove fluid then ultrafiltration via haemodialysis will be needed urgently.

Once the initial overload is corrected then a careful check on the patient's chart should be made. Some patients will apparently be losing 1 or more litres of excess fluid via the dialysis every day, but stay oedematous and do not lose weight. Despite their protestations the only conclusion is that they are drinking too much and their fluid allowance must be reviewed.

However, if there appears to be a genuine problem of fluid removal then leaving the abdomen empty overnight may well be beneficial since in such patients fluid tends to be reabsorbed during long dwell periods. Frusemide can also be tried long-term but may become less effective with time.

Use of all 3.86% bags should not be considered, as paradoxically it may make matters worse, possibly due to dehydration of the peritoneal membrane. Occasionally stopping PD and switching to haemodialysis for a few weeks may allow the abdomen to recover the capacity for ultrafiltration.

If the above measures are not helpful then a permanent change to haemodialysis may be necessary. However recent work suggests that certain pharmacological agents may improve ultrafiltration. Currently verapamil and phosphatidylcholine are the subject of investigation and early results appear promising. Further studies are necessary, though, before they can be recommended for routine clinical use.

Hydrothorax   D

Occasional patients on CAPD develop a large pleural effusion. If they are not grossly overloaded then a leak between the peritoneal and pleural cavities may have occurred. The simplest way of confirming this possibility is to check the pleural fluid glucose. If it is considerably higher than the blood glucose the fluid must be dialysate. Other techniques using isotopes, dyes or radio-opaque media have been described for confirming a leak and locating the site.

Initial treatment should be to stop peritoneal dialysis and aspirate the pleural effusion. The abdomen should be left empty for a period of 1 to 2 weeks and haemodialysis used temporarily. Subsequently peritoneal dialysis can be recommenced with slowly increasing volumes. CAPD should not start until 1 to 2 weeks later. This regime may be sufficient for some patients. If not, a chemical pleurodesis using tetracycline can be tried again with a period off peritoneal dialysis. Alternatively surgical pleurodesis may be necessary. However a change to haemodialysis permanently should be considered when assessing the risks of these procedures.

Oedema of the abdominal wall or genitalia

See the relevant headings in Section A of this manual.

Hypotension   D

The most likely cause of hypotension is excessive fluid loss. This can occur even with CAPD using only 1.36% dextrose. Check the dialysis chart to see the daily fluid recovery. Consistently more than 1 litre excess removed suggests volume depletion as a cause for the hypotension. Look at the daily weight record. If fluid removal has been excessive then the weight will have fallen and the patient should not have any oedema.

Should the patient have been using any 3.86% dextrose then switch to all 1.36% and allow him or her to drink more. This usually corrects the problem. If only 1.36% dextrose has been used increase the daily fluid intake allowance. Occasional patients will need to have intravenous saline to speed recovery.

Examine the patient for other possible causes such as bacteraemia, myocardial infarct, gastro-intestinal bleeding etc.

Should hypotension not be directly related to the dialysis procedure then correct the cause. Continue the dialysis if possible but in the presence of hypotension it is wise to avoid the use of 3.86% dextrose unless there is severe fluid overload.

Hypertension   D

Patients on long-term peritoneal dialysis do not commonly have hypertension. If it does occur then the possibility of fluid overload must be considered. Check for the presence of oedema and see if the daily weight has been rising. Should there be any chance of excess fluid causing the problem increase the number of 3.86% dextrose bags being used in 24 hours. Re-assess the daily fluid intake allowance and re-educate the patient appropriately. As the weight falls blood pressure will usually drop and then the use of 3.86% dextrose can be reduced. Occasional patients will require a hypotensive drug when they have reached their true dry weight.

Dialysis with a stoma   D

It is possible to use a Silastic catheter in an abdomen which has a stoma. However, the risks of infection are greater and if an alternative system of dialysis can be used it should be tried in the first instance. If a Silastic cannula is to be used the skin exit site should be placed as far away as practical from the stoma. Though usually catheters enter the abdomen via the mid-line they can be inserted via the flank if necessary as long as the tunnel is still subcutaneous. As there may be adhesions from the previous operation(s) it is worth considering inserting the cannula under direct vision via a laparotomy.

Peritoneal adhesions and sclerosis   **D**

Long-term peritoneal dialysis is much more difficult if there are adhesions present. Should there be a high chance e.g. there have been several previous laparotomies, it is wiser to have the catheter implanted by a further laparotomy. The surgeon will then be able to assess whether the peritoneal cavity has enough room and is free of sclerosis so that peritoneal dialysis is feasible.

Repeated or prolonged peritonitis may also lead to adhesions making continuation of dialysis difficult. Experience suggests that it is not so much the number of episodes which cause trouble but the length of time the abdomen is inflamed. Fungal infection is notorious for causing adhesions as it may take weeks to clear the abdomen even with amphotericin in the dialysate. To try and reduce the chances of adhesion formation any peritonitis must be treated promptly and vigorously. If the infection is not controlled, judged by clearing of the dialysate outflow, within one week, the catheter should be removed as it is probably contributing to persistence (see section on peritonitis).

Occasionally if a laparotomy is performed on a patient who has had prolonged peritonitis, the peritoneal membrane will be found to have become thick and sclerosed and no longer be a thin shiny structure. Peritoneal dialysis may well have to be abandoned if sclerosis is discovered.

Peritoneal sclerosis may also occur in the absence of recurrent peritonitis. Sometimes a thick tissue cocoons the bowel producing strictures and intestinal obstruction. The exact cause is unclear but it has been associated with the use of acetate in the dialysate and chlorhexidine as an antiseptic for bag changes. Treatment is difficult and recurrent bowel surgery may be necessary. The mortality is high. Prevention at present is confined to using lactate as the buffer in CAPD fluid.

At present it is not certain whether over several years the peritoneal membrane might slowly change with continuing dialysis, especially CAPD, even in the absence of infection. There is some evidence that diabetic patients might have some loss of efficiency of dialysis after a few years possibly due to their microangiopathy. Intermittent peritoneal dialysis or CAPD is certainly possible with success for many years, > 10.

Insertion via laparotomy   D

It is sometimes advisable to implant a Silastic catheter via a laparotomy. This will be necessary for small children and those who may have omental wrapping or if there are doubts about adhesions. After opening the abdomen and if necessary removing the omentum the catheter tip is placed in the pelvis in the recto-vesical or recto-vaginal pouch. The inner cuff is seated above the linea alba as usual and the subcutaneous tunnel constructed in the normal way. The peritoneal incision must be closed carefully avoiding constricting the catheter but tight enough to minimise the chances of hernia formation. The wounds are then closed in a standard manner.

Dialysis after laparotomy   D

Following laparotomy it is important to keep the cannula flushed with a heparin-containing fluid to prevent blockage by clots or fibrin. Dialysis can be recommenced immediately but low volumes must be used to prevent leakage. It is suggested that cycle volumes of one quarter the normal should be used, e.g. 500 ml for an adult normally having 2000 ml cycles. Heparin should be added to the dialysate at a concentration of 500 units per litre. After 2 to 3 days if no problem occurs cycle volumes can be increased to one half, and full amounts used after at least 1 week. If dialysis is not required then the catheter should be flushed by running in 50 ml of heparinised saline every 6 hours. If there are no drains or stomata then a laparotomy wound should be watertight by 48 hours and dialysis can proceed with half size cycle volumes as before.

Hypokalaemia   D

During CAPD a free diet can often be taken, including potassium. Despite this, occasional patients develop hypokalaemia. It is wise to check the actual dietary intake of potassium and ensure it is adequate as patients often stay on their previous chronic renal failure diet, being afraid to change. If this does not solve the problem, oral potassium supplements can be considered or dialysate prescribed containing potassium added by the manufacturer.

Obesity D

Many patients with terminal renal failure are wasted and after starting long-term dialysis will slowly gain dry weight. However, occasional patients having CAPD will become overtly obese. This is related to the absorption of dextrose from the dialysate. It is particularly likely to occur if considerable amounts of 3.86% dextrose are used. If at all possible only one such 'strong' bag should be used per day. Dietary advice should also be given.

Lack of subcutaneous fat D

The standard procedure for inserting a Silastic catheter involves placing the inner cuff just above the linea alba under the subcutaneous fat and then making a tunnel through the fat to the outer cuff which should be at least 2 cm back from the exit site. Occasionally, patients (including small children) are met with little or no fat. Normally the inner cuff is lying nearly vertically above the portion of the catheter going through the peritoneum. However, in patients with no subcutaneous fat it will be found that there is insufficient depth of tissue for the cannula to curve away from the cuff into the tunnel and kinking occurs when closure is attempted. The best solution is to lay the inner cuff on its side and allow the catheter to curve into the peritoneal cavity below this cuff. There will then be no problem in getting the cannula to lie properly in its tunnel.

Backache D

Patients with any form of back trouble may find their symptoms worse when treated with CAPD. This is possibly related to the posture caused by the fluid in the abdomen. Sometimes back exercises and/or a lumbar support may help. Reducing cycle volumes from 2 to 1.5 litres can be considered but the clinician must ensure that the uraemia is still being adequately controlled. Occasionally the only solution is transfer to intermittent peritoneal dialysis or haemodialysis.

Temporary stopping D

Sometimes it is necessary to stop using a Silastic cannula for peritoneal dialysis. This may be because the cannula is blocked or there is a persistent infection either along the cannula track or in the peritoneal cavity itself. This will usually mean the catheter will have to be removed. Dialysis is of course still necessary. It can be continued by either using a temporary PD catheter in the flank or by haemodialysis. The use of a subclavian dialysis system will obviate the need to create shunts which reduce the options for vascular access in the future.

Should the Silastic catheter be merely blocked or require removal for superficial infection it is quite safe to use a temporary PD cannula for continuing dialysis. A new Silastic catheter can then be inserted as soon as the abdomen (both skin and peritoneum) is free of infection. If the initial removal is for continuing peritonitis a temporary PD cannula can be used but if the infection is not controlled as judged by negative cultures and clearing of the fluid within a few days, it is wiser to remove all foreign bodies from the abdomen, give systemic antibiotics and switch to haemodialysis. This is particularly true if fungal peritonitis is present (see section on peritonitis).

A successful transplant will mean the catheter is no longer required. If there is no infection present the cannula may be safely left for some months. It should be aseptically disconnected from the dialysis tubing and then sealed with the rubber cap. If post-operative dialysis is necessary the Silastic catheter can be used for treatment in the normal manner. Sometimes graft function may fail in the first few months. It may be possible to re-establish dialysis using the original catheter. Flushing should be performed prior to connection and if necessary urokinase can be tried. If graft function remains good it is wise to remove the catheter after a few months and thus eliminate a possible source of infection in an immuno-suppressed patient.

Should it be necessary to just stop CAPD for a short period then a 50 ml bag of saline can be used to replace the dialysis fluid bag on the end of the line. This avoids having to disconnect the spike connector. Disconnect caps are available for the end of some types of line. If this procedure is not feasible the line must be removed aseptically and the cannula connector covered with a sterile rubber cap supplied with the catheter. The titanium connector can be sealed quite satisfactorily with this cap.

Hernia   D

One of the recognised complications of CAPD is the development of herniae. These can occur at various sites including through cannula insertion holes, past or present. Herniae commonly become irreducible and may strangulate. It is therefore wise to repair any hernia present prior to starting CAPD.

If a patient develops abdominal pain or a swelling then the possibility of a hernia should be considered. Following repair of any hernia it is important to avoid excessive abdominal distension until the wound is secure in order to minimise the chances of a recurrence. The patient should be changed to intermittent peritoneal dialysis with no dwell time but reduced cycle volumes. 500 ml is recommended for average sized adults. Cycles can be increased to 2 litres over a fortnight and then CAPD may be recommenced. It is wise to add heparin for a few days postoperatively.

Baths, showers, swimming

It is better for patients with a Silastic catheter to have a shower rather than a bath. However, if necessary, the bag and tubing can be hung over the side of the bath. Following washing, the area around the cannula exit is dried, cleansed with povidone-iodine and dressed as described in the section on exit site care.

Swimming is feasible. The empty bag with the rolled up tubing should be placed inside a thin plastic bag, e.g. a freezer bag, and a rubber band or freezer bag tie placed around the neck tightly to reduce the entry of water. Both males and females should wear a full-length swimming costume rather than trunks or bikinis. This merely makes it easier to stow away the system under the costume and avoids having too many onlookers staring or even complaining about contamination! After swimming the exit site is dried and dressed as before. The dressing or shield around the bag and tubing connection should also be renewed.

If repeated swimming is likely, e.g. on holiday, then stoma adhesive should be placed around the exit site and then covered with a stoma ring. The empty bag and line can be placed in a clip-on stoma bag while swimming. This should provide a watertight seal for the holiday period.

Patients who have a disconnect system, e.g. Baxter O set or Freeline, will have little problem in disguising their cannula and will need no special measures whilst swimming.

Use of insulin   D

Increased numbers of diabetic patients with renal failure are being treated by peritoneal dialysis. Those who are receiving intermittent peritoneal dialysis, manual or by machine, will need to have an increased dose of insulin to cover the glucose load during the procedure. It is advisable to give the insulin just prior to starting dialysis. The exact dose has to be determined for each patient. As a starting point it is suggested the usual dose is increased by 4 units whether a short or long acting preparation is prescribed. Blood glucose should be checked 2 hourly using the paper test strips with occasional laboratory estimations. The dose can then be regulated for the next dialysis. Once a suitable regime has been found, unless the patient becomes ill for some other reason, the insulin dosage will not need changing.

Patients having CAPD can have their insulin administered intra-peritoneally. The majority of dialysis units inject the drug into the bag just prior to inflow. The dose necessary for control will be considerably higher than that required subcutaneously. Only short acting insulin is used. Patients should first be established on CAPD and control of their diabetes maintained by parenteral drug. The total number of units used in 24 hours is calculated and this figure is increased by 50%. This final result is divided by four to give the starting doses of insulin to be used for the first four cycles. The morning parenteral dose of insulin is omitted and the increased amount is given in the first bag. Blood sugars are checked 2 hourly by paper stick with occasional laboratory confirmation. Doses can be increased daily as necessary. A further increase may be necessary for 3.86% dextrose bags. The insulin should be added via the injection port on the bag (Figure B10). Immediately after the drug has been administered, inflow should start.

If at all possible any diabetic patient on dialysis (or a family member) should be taught to check the blood glucose by finger-prick and paper strip testing, preferably with the aid of a meter.

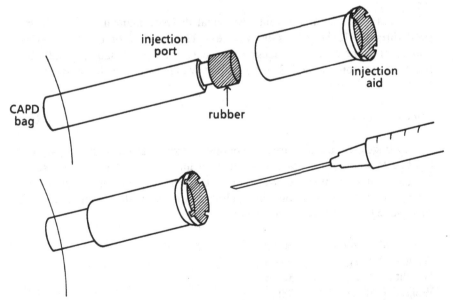

Figure B10 Use of injection aid. The metal injection aid fits over the injection port. Its funnel-shaped end guides the needle into the rubber injection port

Insulin drawn up in a syringe is stable in a refrigerator for up to 24 hours. If the patient is unable to draw up the drug him or herself then a helper or a nurse can prepare all four doses first thing in the morning and leave them in separate syringes laid out in order in the fridge to keep cool. Even blind patients can then usually be taught to add the injection to the bag, if necessary utilizing a metal sleeve which fits over the injection port and is shaped to guide the needle into the rubber (Figure B10).

How many cycles?   D

Most of the data available regarding the long-term clinical use of CAPD has been obtained on patients using four cycles in 24 hours. A few centres have tried three cycles per day and good results are claimed. It is probable that children need relatively more dialysis than adults if there is to be the maximum chance of growth so four cycles are definitely recommended. However, it is permissible for any patient to miss one bag change in order to have a day out as long as this does not happen too frequently. Patients who have a fluid overload problem will definitely be better on four rather than three cycles a day. Patients able to tolerate 2500 ml cycles may only require three cycles a day.

Patients having intermittent peritoneal dialysis, manual or by machine, need three 10-12 hour sessions a week. The number of cycles is not so important as the volume exchanged per week. For a 70 kg man up to 120 litres per week is recommended. Smaller patients will need proportionately less.

Choice of volume   D

CAPD bags are manufactured to contain less dialysate than the capacity of the bag to allow room for excess fluid during outflow. It is best to use the biggest volume compatible with comfort. Some patients may feel bloated when switched to CAPD but this feeling disappears with continuing dialysis. As a guide the following is suggested:

Very small children	-	300 ml
Weight 10-20 kg	-	500 ml
Weight 20-30 kg	-	1000 ml
Weight 30-50 kg	-	1500 ml
Weight > 50 kg	-	2000 ml

Some bigger patients may tolerate 2500 ml cycles and may then be able to reduce to three cycles a day.

Automatic machine PD allows cycle volume to be adjusted for each individual but once again most adults should have a 2 litre cycle.

Choice of antiseptic   **D**

Povidone-iodine is the agent of choice. If, however, the patient is genuinely allergic to the compound then hydrogen peroxide can be used for cleansing cannula exit sites and alcohol can be used for connection and disconnection points.

Heating the fluid

Heating of CAPD fluid is not absolutely essential but greatly improves patient comfort. Dry heat is essential and the bags should be warm to touch but not hot. Flat plate bag warmers are commercially available though not all are electrically safe. Microwave ovens have been suggested but in Britain the Departments of Health have strongly advised against their usage as bags have ruptured due to uneven heating. At home an airing cupboard is often satisfactory. In hospital a laboratory type incubator is most satisfactory for multiple patient use (see section A). All CCPD systems incorporate a heater.

Wet heat must never be used because of the risk of infection.

Suggested Further Reading

1. Tenckhoff, H. (1974). *Chronic Peritoneal Dialysis* (Seattle: University of Washington)
2. Nolph, K.D. (1981). *Peritoneal Dialysis*, 2nd Edn. (The Hague: Martinus Nijhoff)
3. *Peritoneal Dialysis Bulletin*, edited by D.G. Oreopoulous, Toronto (Quarterly. Official journal of the International Society for Peritoneal Dialysis)
4. Gokal, R. (1986). *Continuous Ambulatory Peritoneal Dialysis*. (Edinburgh: Churchill Livingstone)
5. Keane, W.F., Everett, E.D., Fine, R.N., Golper, T.A., Vas, S.I. and Peterson, P.K. (1987). CAPD-related peritonitis management and antibiotic therapy recommendations. *Peritoneal Dialysis Bulletin*, 7, 55-68
6. Working party of the British Society for Antimicrobial Chemotherapy. (1987). Diagnosis and management of peritonitis in continuous ambulatory peritoneal dialysis. *Lancet*, 1, 845-849
7. Oreopoulos, D.G. *et al.* (1987). Peritoneal catheters and exit site practices: current recommendations. *Peritoneal Dialysis Bulletin*, 7, 130-138

Index

Note: In the text, *cannula* and *catheter* have been used interchangeably. In the index, *catheter* has been used throughout.